Managing Chronic Health Needs in Child Care and Schools

A QUICK REFERENCE GUIDE

Editors

Elaine A. Donoghue, MD, FAAP

Colleen A. Kraft, MD, FAAP

American Academy of Pediatrics

141 Northwest Point Blvd

Elk Grove Village, IL 60007-1098

American Academy of Pediatrics Department of Marketing and Publications Staff

Maureen DeRosa, MPA
Director, Department of Marketing and Publications

Mark Grimes
Director, Division of Product Development

Jeff Mahony
Manager, Product Development

Eileen Glasstetter
Manager, Product Development

Mark Ruthman
Manager, Electronic Product Development

Sandi King, MS
Director, Division of Publishing and Production Services

Jason Crase
Editorial Specialist

Leesa Levin-Doroba
Manager, Publishing and Production Services

Peg Mulcahy
Manager, Graphic Design and Production

Jill Ferguson
Director, Division of Marketing

Linda Smessaert
Manager, Clinical and Professional Publications Marketing

Robert Herling
Director, Division of Sales

Library of Congress Control Number: 2009924069
ISBN: 978-1-58110-299-4
MA0443

The recommendations in this publication do not indicate an exclusive course of treatment or serve as a standard of medical care. Variations, taking into account individual circumstances, may be appropriate.

Brand names are furnished for identification purposes only. Inclusion in this publication does not imply endorsement.
The American Academy of Pediatrics (AAP) does not recommend any specific brand of products or services. Listing of resources does not imply endorsement by the AAP. The AAP is not responsible for the content of the resources mentioned in this publication. Phone numbers and Web site addresses are as current as possible, but may change at any time.

For permission to reproduce material from this publication, visit www.copyright.com and search for Managing Chronic Health Needs in Child Care and Schools.

9-247/Rep0914   5 6 7 8 9 10

Reviewers/Contributors

Editors

Elaine A. Donoghue, MD, FAAP
Colleen A. Kraft, MD, FAAP

Contributors

Abbey Alkon, RN, PhD
Judy Calder, RN, MS
Angela Crowley, PhD, APRN, PNP-BC, FAAN
Linda M. Grant, MD, MPH, FAAP

Technical Reviewers

Wendy K. Anderson, MD, FAAP
Susan S. Aronson, MD, FAAP
Robert Burke, MD, FAAP
Linda M. Grant, MD, MPH, FAAP
Barbara U. Hamilton, MA
Patti Lucarelli, RN, MSN, CPNP, APN
Linda K. Smith

Reviewers

Thomas C. Abshire, MD, FAAP
Robert D. Baker, Jr, MD, FAAP
Robert Beekman, MD, FAAP
Drucy S. Borowitz, MD, FAAP
Michael T. Brady, MD, FAAP
Stuart Brink, MD, FAAP
Marilyn J. Bull, MD, FAAP
William J. Byrne, MD, FAAP
William L. Clarke, MD, FAAP
Ellen Roy Elias, MD, FAAP
Stephen A. Feig, MD, FAAP
Paul Fisher, MD, FAAP
Joseph T. Flynn, MD, MS, FAAP

John Foreman, MD, FAAP
Robert W. Frenck, Jr, MD, FAAP
Frank Galioto, MD, FAAP
Laura Hoyt, MD, FAAP
Chris Plauché Johnson, MD, MEd, FAAP
Julie Katkin, MD, FAAP
Howard W. Kilbride, MD, FAAP
Mitchell R. Lester, MD, FAAP
Donald Lewis, MD, FAAP
Gregory Liptak, MD, FAAP
Michael I. Reiff, MD, FAAP
Howard M. Saal, MD, FAAP
Robert A. Saul, MD, FAAP

Janet Silverstein, MD, FAAP
Donny W. Suh, MD, FAAP
Howard Taras, MD, FAAP
Milton Tenenbein, MD, FAAP
Steven J. Wassner, MD, FAAP
Eric J. Werner, MD, FAAP
Lani Wheeler, MD, FAAP
Susan Wiley, MD, FAAP
Russell Van Dyke, MD, FAAP
Beth A. Vogt, MD, FAAP
Jeanette Zaichkin, RN, MN-NNP-BC

American Academy of Pediatrics

Errol R. Alden, MD, FAAP
Executive Director/CEO

Roger F. Suchyta, MD, FAAP
Associate Executive Director

Maureen DeRosa, MPA
Director, Department of Marketing and Publications

Mark Grimes
Director, Division of Product Development

Jeff Mahony
Manager, Product Development

Fan Tait, MD, FAAP
Associate Executive Director/Director, Department of Community and Specialty Pediatrics

Jeanne M. Anderson, MEd
Manager, Early Education and Child Care Initiatives

Madra Guinn-Jones, MPH
Manager, Committees and Sections

Additional AAP Staff
Eileen Glasstetter
Renee Jarrett
Stephanie Nelson, MS, CHES
Mark Ruthman

I was inspired to write this book by the many people who taught me the importance of loving care and respect in the development of a strong person, with or without special needs. I would like to dedicate this book to my father, John J. Donoghue; my brother, Robert Donoghue; and to all of my family who supported me. Thank you also to my mentors and colleagues at the American Academy of Pediatrics.

— Elaine A. Donoghue, MD, FAAP

This book is a sampling of wisdom gained during my interwoven professions of pediatrician and parent. These lessons were learned from my family, especially my children, Daniel, Julie, and Tim Kraft; from Patsy Moon and the Child Development Center at the Medical College of Virginia, whom I credit for my practical knowledge in early care and education; from my mentors both in pediatric practice and at the American Academy of Pediatrics; and from my families, who teach me daily about what really matters in caring for children with special health care needs. We would like to thank the people who contributed to writing and reviewing this book.

— Colleen A. Kraft, MD, FAAP

Table of Contents

Introduction:
Safe and Appropriate
Care of Children With
Chronic Health Needs

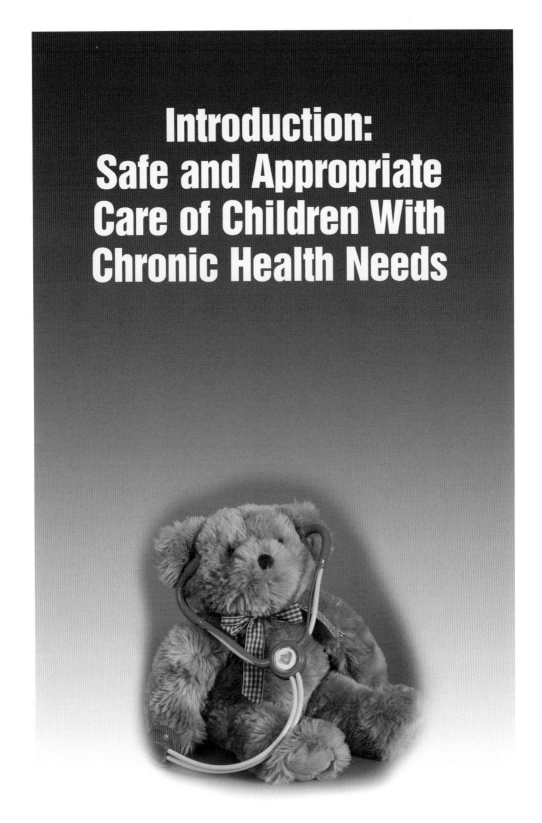

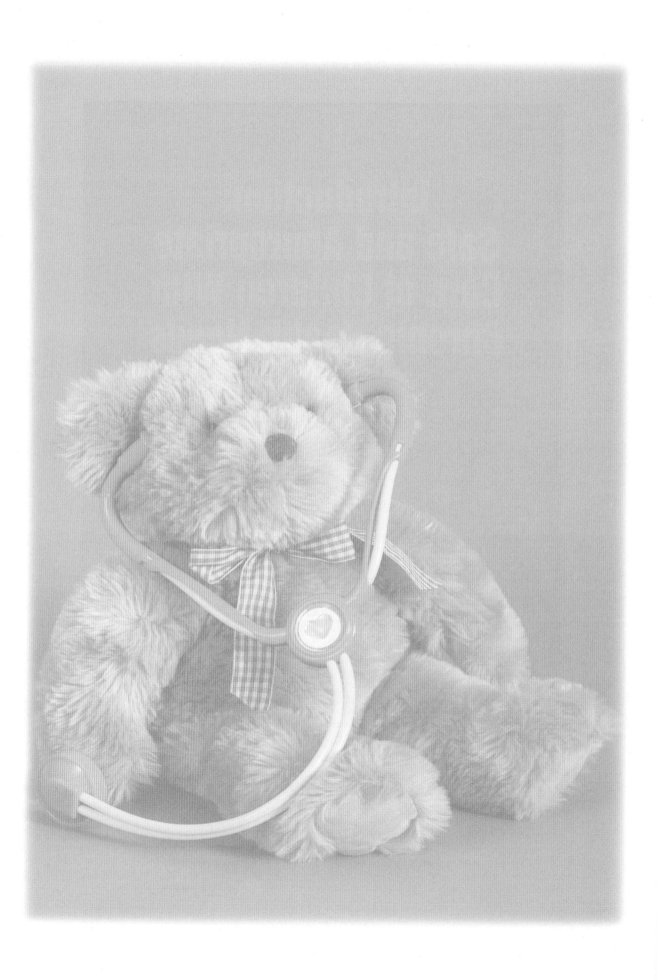

Introduction: Safe and Appropriate Care of Children With Chronic Health Needs

Large numbers of children have chronic medical conditions or special health care needs. In fact, federal data from the large *National Survey of Children with Special Health Care Needs Chartbook 2005–2006* (US Department of Health and Human Services, 2008) show that 14% of all children in this country have special health care needs. This federal survey defined children with special health care needs as "…those who have or are at increased risk for a chronic physical, developmental, behavioral, or emotional condition and who also require health and related services of a type or amount beyond that required by children generally" (*Pediatrics.* 1998;102:137–140). This study helped us to understand that special health care needs are common and that the spectrum of needs is broad.

The miracles of modern medicine have helped many children survive what might have been lethal illnesses in the past, but many times parents and children are left with challenges in maintaining their health, well-being, and quality of life. Children are living longer and healthier lives with medical conditions, and they can participate in activities that would have been unthinkable in the past.

This book was written to address the fact that children are often in out-of-home settings for a large portion of their day as they attend school, child care, and recreational programs. Many school-aged children have access to a school nurse to help with their medical needs, even if that nurse is only available on an intermittent basis. Preschool children, infants, toddlers, and children in before- and after-school care seldom have the benefit of an on-site health professional like the school nurse. For the youngest children this lack of access to professional health oversight is ironic because these children often have more frequent illnesses and are less able to verbalize their needs. Schools face different challenges because their mandate to provide education under federal funding results in a different set of guidelines.

The needs of children with chronic medical conditions and special health care needs vary with age and increasing independence. Regardless, the need for resources and strategies to help caregivers/teachers face the challenges of caring for children with chronic medical conditions and special health care needs is undeniable.

It is vital to bridge the communication gap between caregivers/teachers and health care professionals so they can work together to mobilize resources and strategies to benefit children and families in their care. Users of this book may include those who work in schools and early childhood

From the Editors About the Book Title

The health conditions described in this book cover a spectrum of chronic illnesses, acute situations, selected developmental and behavioral problems, and special health care needs, with a special emphasis on children with special health care needs. For this reason, we chose the broad title, *Managing Chronic Health Needs in Child Care and Schools: A Quick Reference Guide,* to emphasize the inclusive nature of the subjects covered, including many common conditions that caregivers/teachers deal with on a daily basis.

programs such as teachers, administrators, school nurses, and caregivers. We also hope that the medical community will use this book to help to communicate a child's chronic medical conditions or special health care needs clearly.

Physicians face numerous requests to complete medical forms for children, but they often have difficulty translating the child's medical needs into practical information that caregivers/teachers need to know. This creates frustration as caregivers/teachers attempt to get appropriate information from busy doctors, many times with the parent as an intermediary. Uncertainty related to privacy laws and rules confound this problem.

The goal of this book is to provide a quick reference that addresses a variety of common chronic health problems that children face. Our guiding question is, "What are the most important things that this caregiver/teacher needs to know for the safe and appropriate care of this child?"

Overview

- Background: Chapter 2 will give a brief background of the services and systems that support care of children with chronic medical conditions and special health care needs.
- The treatment team: Doctors, therapists, specialists, families, caregivers/teachers, school nurses; the team that supports the child is wonderful, but the roles team members play can be confusing. Chapter 3 will outline who the team members can be and what role they play. The medical home will also be discussed.

- Care Plans: The Care Plan is the blueprint for caring for children with chronic medical conditions and special health care needs. Chapter 4 will review different types of Care Plans and what they include.
- Implementing the Care Plan: Chapters 5, 6, and 8 will discuss methods to implement a Care Plan, especially when it includes administering medication or preparing for an emergency. Many children, such as those with life-threatening allergies, function normally, but they need special planning for emergencies.
- New conditions or signs of concern: This book is designed to address a child who already has a diagnosis, but the reality is that many children will develop a medical problem while they are in out-of-home care. Chapter 7 addresses what signs are worrisome and how to address those concerns with families.
- The second half of the book consists of condition-specific Quick Reference Sheets. Remember that each child is an individual, not a disease or a disorder. Most diseases and disorders have a wide range of severity. One child with spina bifida may walk and another might require a wheelchair. The Quick Reference Sheets are designed to point out what *might* be a problem for a child with that condition. The child's individual Care Plan will outline what is true for that *specific* child.

A short Quick Reference Sheet can only scratch the surface of many medical conditions. There is a wealth of material in print, on video, and on the Internet; however, not all of this information is accurate. The Web site for the American Academy of Pediatrics, www.aap.org, is an excellent starting point for reliable information. The resources at the end of each Quick Reference Sheet and in Additional Resources will be a guide to further trustworthy sources of information.

Caregivers/teacher can play a very important role in the life of children with chronic medical conditions and special health care needs. Caring for these children can provide an opportunity to teach all children about respect, helping others, and including those with differences. Children with chronic health needs sometimes can feel that their condition is "their fault"; they need reassurance that this is not true. They need support in dealing with their challenges and reminders of their strengths. It can be inspiring for all to see how a child with a chronic medical condition or special need adapts to face this challenge. Parents also benefit from watching their child gain independence and learn new skills. In addition, parents can benefit from the support that a teacher or caregiver can provide.

Caring for children with chronic medical conditions and special health care needs can be challenging, but the rewards can be enormous for the children, their families, their health professionals, and their caregivers/teachers.

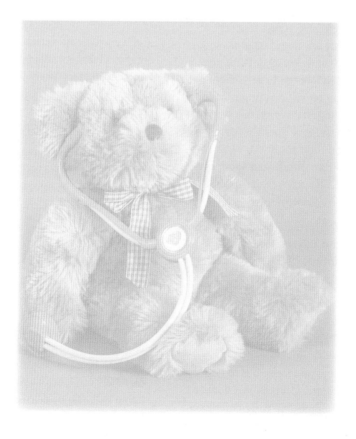

CHAPTER 2

Background

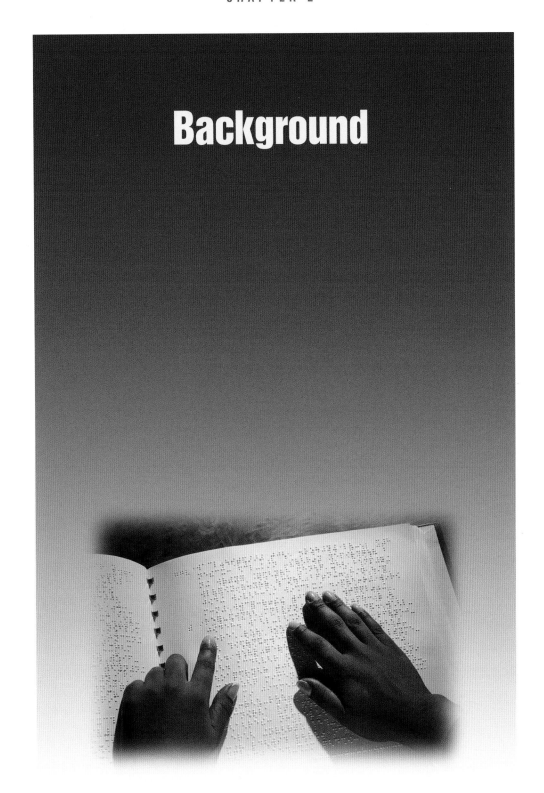

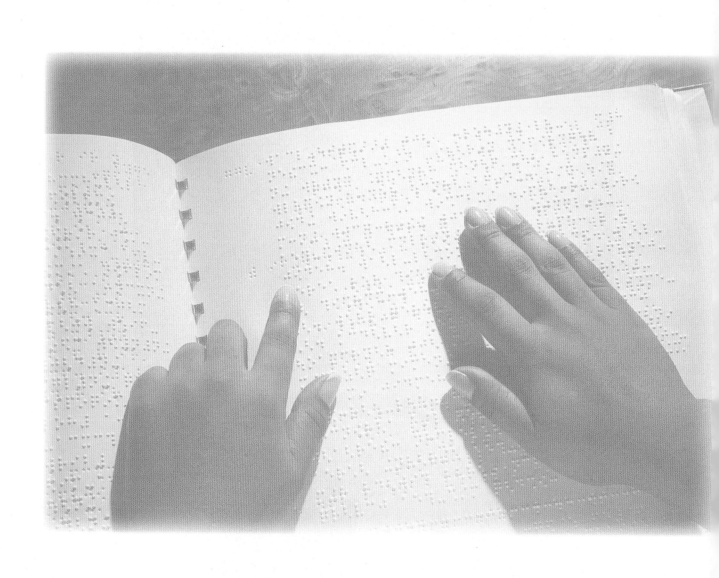

Background

Families, Health Professionals, and Child Care/Schools: A Three-Way Communication

Parents of children with chronic medical conditions and special health care needs share the same joys, challenges, and concerns that other parents have with their children. Once their children make contact with the health care system, these parents start communicating with medical and therapy providers. Their children often receive care from different kinds of doctors and other health care professionals—primary care specialists and pediatric subspecialists. They may see an occupational therapist, a physical therapist, a speech/language therapist, or a counselor to receive care for their condition. Caregivers/teachers for these young children may have questions about the recommendations provided by these health professionals, which may include daily routines, a child's medication, medical equipment, or behavior management.

The prime mandate of school districts is to provide a quality education. The caregiving responsibility of school districts exists within the context of the educational mission. The caregiving focus is on managing safety during school hours as well as ensuring that the child receives the appropriate accommodations to academically achieve at his or her highest level. Schools are, financially and otherwise, responsible for space, equipment, and personnel required to meet student needs if the needs are determined to interfere with learning, school attendance, or access to school programs. Correct placement in the least restrictive environment is central to a school educational mission. Presence of a full-time school nurse, accessible buildings, nurse practice laws, union rules, and state regulations will affect how a school can provide the appropriate accommodations for safety and academic achievement.

To be effectively involved in the child's care, child care professionals and school personnel need to communicate with a child's parents as well as important medical and therapy professionals who are making recommendations for the care of the child. This quick reference guide will discuss the use of a Care Plan, an important written document that fosters communication among all those involved with a child. Three-way communication that involves the family, the child's other caregivers/teachers, and the child's health professionals enables collaboration among all team members, asking and answering questions that facilitate the best experience for a child.

Here's an example—the parents of a child with a seizure disorder enroll the child at a child care center. The pediatric neurologist caring for the child communicates to the parents/guardians the type and dose of medication necessary to keep this child healthy. If the child care professionals have received training on how to give medication safely, often it is the parent who provides information to the caregivers/teachers about how to have the child accept this medication most readily, which of the foods that are OK to use work best for mixing, and tips for ensuring that the child will take all of this medication. Even though the neurologist's phone information is available for emergencies and the neurologist has indicated the circumstances that require a call, it is the parent who will often advise child care professionals on triggers for this child's seizures.

Three-way communication among parents, medical professionals, and others who are responsible for children during the day promotes optimal care for a child with chronic medical conditions or special health care needs. This communication among all partners should recognize, value, and make use of the opportunity for collaboration among the members of the child's team.

Individuals With Disabilities Education Act (IDEA)

The Individuals With Disabilities Education Act (IDEA) requires states and localities to provide education and related services (eg, physical or speech therapy) to infants, toddlers, children, and youth with disabilities. The history of IDEA reflects our changing attitude as a society toward children with disabilities.

Prior to the 1970s many children with conditions such as Down syndrome or autism resided in institutions. Over time, many parents and professionals recognized the benefits to these children and their families of living at home, in their communities. As these children entered the school systems within their localities, laws were developed to help meet their individual needs. Congress enacted the Education for All Handicapped Children Act (Public Law 94-142) in 1975.

There were 4 purposes of Public Law 94-142.
- To ensure that all children with disabilities have available to them a free appropriate public education that emphasizes special education and related services designed to meet their unique needs.
- To ensure that the rights of children with disabilities and their parents are protected.

- To assist states and localities to provide for the education of all children with disabilities.
- To assess and ensure the effectiveness of efforts to educate all children with disabilities.

Public Law 94-142 was a response to congressional concern for 2 groups of children—the more than 1 million children with disabilities who were *excluded entirely* from the education system, and those who had only *limited access* to the education system and were therefore denied an appropriate education. This latter group comprised more than half of all children with disabilities who were living in the United States at that time. These issues of improved access became guiding principles for further advances in educating children with disabilities over the last quarter of the 20th century.

Over the next few decades, this law was amended to provide services to children and youth with health impairments. Hearing, vision, orthopedic, and developmental disabilities can clearly affect a child's educational ability, and IDEA seeks to develop supports that accommodate all children as individuals. Today, IDEA provides services to infants and toddlers through *early intervention* (Part C of IDEA). Children 3 years and older are served through *special education and related services* (Part B of IDEA).

Early Intervention (Part C of IDEA)

Early intervention (Part C of IDEA) is the process of providing services, education, and support to young children (birth through 36 months) who are found to have any of the following:
- A diagnosed physical or mental condition with a high probability of resulting in a developmental delay.
- An existing delay per a state's criteria for eligibility.
- A risk of developing a delay or special need that may affect development or impede education. (This at-risk category depends on the state's eligibility determination process and whether it includes children who are at risk. States are given the discretion of including children at risk in their state plans.)

Part C of IDEA was established in recognition of "an urgent and substantial need" to
- Enhance the development of infants and toddlers with disabilities.
- Reduce educational costs by minimizing the need for special education through early intervention.
- Minimize the likelihood of institutionalization and maximize independent living.
- Enhance the capacity of families to meet their child's needs.

The purpose of early intervention is to provide the therapy and support that will allow a child to "catch up," so that by preschool age, the child can function at the level of age-appropriate peers. For children with developmental delay who will require therapy along the continuum of their life, early intervention can significantly reduce the adverse effects of their disability or delay. Services are designed to identify and meet a child's needs in the following 5 developmental areas: physical development, cognitive development, communication, social and emotional development, and adaptive development.

Early intervention programs and services may occur in a variety of settings, with a heavy emphasis on *natural environments.* By definition, natural environments mean "settings that are natural or normal for the child's age peers who have no disabilities" (34 CFR §303.18). Part C of IDEA requires that "to the maximum extent appropriate to the needs of the child, early intervention services must be provided in natural environments, including the home and community settings in which children without disabilities participate" (34 CFR §303.12[b]). For this reason, it is important for caregivers/teachers to understand basic principles about inclusion and children with chronic medical conditions and special health care needs. The provision of early intervention services taking place in natural environments is not just a suggestion; it is a legal requirement.

The exception to the natural environments rule reads, "The provision of early intervention services for any infant or toddler with a disability occurs in a setting other than a natural environment that is most appropriate, as determined by the parent and the Individualized Family Service Plan (IFSP) team, only when early intervention cannot be achieved satisfactorily for the infant or toddler in a natural environment."

Early intervention services are proven to be most effective when started as soon as the child's delay or disability is identified. A therapist or an educator may be assigned to a child in the group setting. There can be many advantages to this; caregivers/teachers may learn tips from the therapist to use with other children and situations for which that caregiver/teacher is responsible. For example, the caregiver/teacher may work with a speech therapist to target goals for a child with speech delay, and learn some exercises that will promote improved speech skills for all the children in the group!

The process of determining and following a child through early intervention has 5 components.
- Child Find
- Evaluation and Assessment
- Eligibility for Part C of IDEA
- Individualized Family Service Plan
- Transitioning Out of Part C of IDEA and Into Part B of IDEA (Special Education)

Child Find

Child Find is a component of IDEA that requires states to identify, locate, and evaluate all children with disabilities, aged birth to 21 years, who are in need of early intervention or special education services. Anyone, including a parent, caregiver, teacher, nurse, or physician, can make a referral to Child Find. After referral, a child will be screened and evaluated if the screening demonstrates a probability of delay. If you think that a child might have a developmental delay, the first step might be to suggest that the parent call Child Find to ask to have the child screened. This process is different from state to state; some states may use a screening phone call to determine the need for further evaluation. Other states may screen a child in a face-to-face meeting with the child's family.

Evaluation and Assessment

Under IDEA, evaluation and assessments are to be provided at no cost to the parent. *Evaluation* refers to the process used by the multidisciplinary team (qualified people with training and experience in the areas of speech and language skills, physical abilities, hearing and vision, and other important areas of development) to find out whether the child is eligible for early intervention services. As part of the evaluation, the multidisciplinary team will observe, interact, and use other tools or methods to gather information on a child. These procedures will help the team find out how the child functions. The team will then meet with the parents/guardians to discuss whether the findings mean that the child is eligible for services under Part C of IDEA.

Eligibility for Part C of IDEA

Eligibility defines if a child demonstrates enough delay to need early intervention. Eligibility is determined by each state's definition of developmental delay and whether it includes children at risk for disabilities. An important part of the evaluation process for infants and toddlers (aged 0–36 months) includes informed clinical opinion of professionals experienced with the development of very young children. States have been given a lot of discretion for determining eligibility for entry into their programs. If the child is determined to be eligible, the next step is to create a plan to address the child's needs, called an IFSP.

Individualized Family Service Plan

An IFSP is the written document that guides the early intervention process for children with disabilities and their families. Effective early intervention is implemented through the IFSP in accordance with Part C of IDEA. It contains information about the services necessary to enhance a child's development and promote the family's involvement to help the child's development. Through the IFSP process, family members and service providers work as a team to plan, implement, and evaluate services specific to the family's concerns, priorities, and available resources. A service coordinator then helps the family by coordinating the services outlined in the IFSP.

Transitioning Out of Part C of IDEA and Into Part B of IDEA (Special Education)

Some children will continue to need services to accommodate their disabilities or enhance their learning beyond 36 months of age. At this age, a child may transition into a special education, or Part B of IDEA, program. Your team (including parents/guardians) should start preparing the child for transition into Part B services around the age of 30 to 32 months (and no later than 3 months prior to the child's third birthday). Not all children will be eligible to enter into preschool special education programs. If it is determined that the child will need special education services, a transition planning meeting will be held to discuss next steps, particularly how to prepare the child for the transition out of Part C of IDEA. During this process, the child will have a new Individualized Education Program (IEP), developed to help continue the child's learning.

Many children who enter the early intervention program master their skills and are able to "graduate." This graduation may occur at any age, as long as the child has met the goals set out by the team.

Special Education and Related Services (Part B of IDEA)

Children may obtain special education and related services through the school system, which is Part B of IDEA. Many children who attend child care enter Part B from early intervention. Others enter the system once a disability is identified after they reach 3 years of age.

The evaluation for special education and related services is multidisciplinary, much like early intervention. The information gathered from the evaluation is used to decide
- If a child is eligible for special education and related services (ie, if they have a disability that will affect their education)
- The services that the school can provide to meet a child's educational needs

Note that services are provided through Part B of IDEA solely to meet a child's educational needs. Under IDEA, parents/guardians are included in the group that decides a child's eligibility for special education services. If a child is found eligible for special education services under IDEA, parents/guardians will work with the school to design an IEP.

The Individuals With Disabilities Education Act Amendments of 1997 list 13 disability categories. A child can be found eligible to receive special education and related services under the following categories:

- Autism
- Deafness
- Deaf-blindness
- Hearing impairment
- Intellectual disability
- Multiple disabilities
- Orthopedic impairment
- Other health impairment
- Serious emotional disturbance
- Specific learning disability
- Speech or language impairment
- Traumatic brain injury
- Visual impairment, including blindness

What Are Related Services?

The regulations in IDEA define the term *related services* as "transportation and such developmental, corrective, and other supportive services as are required to assist a child with a disability to benefit from special education…" (Section 300.24[a]). The following are included within the definition of related services:

- Speech-language pathology and audiology services
- Psychological services
- Physical and occupational therapies
- Recreation, including therapeutic recreation
- Early identification and assessment of disabilities in children
- Counseling services, including rehabilitation counseling
- Orientation and mobility services
- Medical services for diagnostic or evaluation purposes
- School health services
- Social work services in schools
- Parent counseling and training
- Transportation

Where Are Related Services Provided?

In recent years, there has been a significant shift in *where* related services are provided. Rather than providing services in a separate room, as was the common practice in years past, schools are emphasizing the provision of some services to students in natural activities and environments. This could include wherever the child's usual activities are.

Today it is not unusual to find speech-language services integrated into instructional activities in any activity area in the group setting. Occupational or physical therapy may be provided during indoor or outdoor active play at a preschool. Usually the therapist will work with teachers and parents/

guardians to shape activities in the curriculum that promote the goals of that child's IEP. For example, a goal for a child with a physical disability may be learning to maneuver a playground without injury; in this case, a physical therapist may work with a caregiver/teacher to help this child gain competence with climbing up a sliding board ladder. The playground serves as the appropriate educational venue for pursing this child's goal!

An IEP should address the child's strengths and the challenges presented by the particular disability. The goals, objectives, and accommodations in a child's IEP are determined to help that child succeed in school.

Special Needs in Grades K Through 12

Children with chronic medical conditions and special health care needs may also have special education needs, depending on the disability. Three major laws affect the provision of services to students with special health care needs. These laws classify disabilities differently, depending on whether it is the Americans With Disabilities Act (ADA), Section 504 of the Rehabilitation Act of 1973, or IDEA. The distinction takes on more significance within the K through 12 years. In the ADA, children are classified as disabled if they have a condition that severely limits daily activities of life. Section 504 defines *disability* as a "mental or physical limitation that substantially limits one or more major life activities" and covers students requiring certain modifications to access education. However, IDEA focuses on disability as one of 13 conditions that handicap *educational* achievement. There is significant overlap among all of these definitions. The services a child receives depends on the disability and its relation to academic impairment.

Under IDEA, if the school team determines that the disability meets the criteria and that the disability adversely affects academic performance, the child is eligible for special education. Under Section 504, if the student meets the eligibility requirements as a "disabled person," he or she is eligible for accommodations that enable the student to have an education comparable to that of a student who is not disabled. It is not a requirement that the disability affects educational performance, and special education may not be required. Section 504 is an antidiscrimination act that extends the educational rights of students with disabilities to private schools. There are no federal funds available, making schools and school districts responsible for funding the reasonable modifications and accommodations in the regular classroom setting as required under Section 504. Children with chronic medical conditions and special health care needs can belong to one or both of these categories. They may be in special education and have an IEP, or they may be in regular education with accommodations provided by a Section 504 plan. Both plans ensure that the child receives a free and appropriate education in the least restrictive environment.

A child may also have chronic medical conditions or special health care needs but not have a Section 504 plan or an IEP. It is possible for there to be accommodations outside of an official Section 504 plan for a child in regular education. Unlike IDEA, under which the school district receives funding for eligible students to provide the related services, Section 504 does not provide any additional funds to assist in accommodating the disability. Nevertheless, the school district is obligated to provide reasonable accommodations.

The No Child Left Behind Act of 2001 (NCLB) was enacted to support elementary and secondary education. The reauthorization of IDEA in 2004 made changes to align itself more effectively with sections of NCLB. These changes focus on the academic achievement role of schools more than the safety component.

See Additional Resources (page 197) for more information.

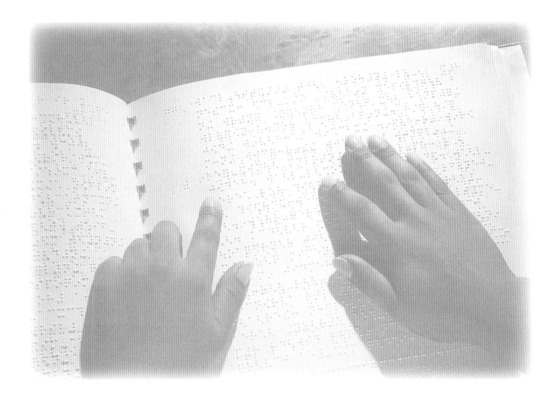

CHAPTER 3

The Treatment Team: Partners in Caring for Children With Chronic Health Needs

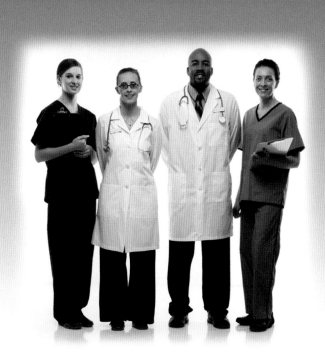

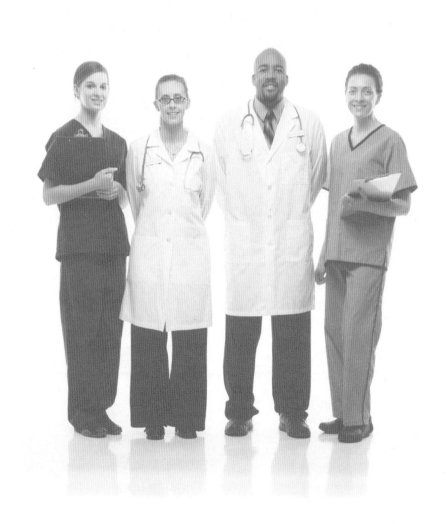

The Treatment Team: Partners in Caring for Children With Chronic Health Needs

The saying, "It takes a village to raise a child," is very true when caring for a child with chronic medical conditions or special health care needs. The core team always includes the parents/guardians of the child, the health care professional in the medical home, and those who are responsible for the care and education of the child during some part of the child's day—child care providers and teachers. Other team members can be very valuable in helping coordinate and implement the plan.

See Chapter 4 for details of roles for each of these participants.

Core Team

Parent/guardian	Knows the child best and can give valuable information.
Health care professional	Completes the Care Plan with input of involved health professionals.
Child care providers/ teachers/ school nurse	Implement the Care Plan.

Other Team Members

Therapists (physical, occupational, speech)	May give therapy sessions while the child attends child care/school. Can suggest adaptations to help the child's functioning. Often part of the Individualized Education Program or Individualized Family Service Plan (see Chapter 2 for more information).
Respiratory therapist	May be helpful to teach staff how to use nebulizers or other equipment to help breathing.
Child care health consultants	Many are health professionals, frequently registered nurses with special training in providing consultation in early education and child care settings, who can help give practical Care Plan implementation tips.
Pediatric subspecialists	These physicians have special expertise in particular health problems or body systems. Sometimes they may act as primary care providers for children with complex health conditions.
Counselors	These mental health professionals can help children with mental health or behavioral needs.
Social workers	Can help connect families to helpful resources.
Registered dietitians/nutritionists	Professionals with special training in food, food preparation, and feeding, and how these aspects of food relate to health, can help with children's dietary needs.
Pharmacists	Professionals with specialized knowledge about medications may be helpful in addressing issues of types, doses, storage, administration, and disposal of medications.
Medical equipment suppliers	May be helpful in teaching staff how to use and maintain medical equipment.

Role of the Health Consultant

All child care and school settings should have access to a health professional who provides consultation and technical assistance on health issues. In schools, this is usually a school nurse. Child care facilities often do not have an on-site health professional, but they can request child care health consultation from professionals with special expertise in topics as they relate to child care such as infectious diseases, nutrition, socio-emotional development, emergency management, and injury prevention. The path for locating a health consultant varies from state to state. For more information, contact your local Child Care Resource & Referral Agency (CCR&R) or the Healthy Child Care Consultant Network (http://hcccnsc.edc.org), or visit www.healthychildcare.org.

Role of Therapists

Many children with developmental delays benefit from therapy to help them develop their skills to the best of their abilities and to learn techniques to adapt to their limitations. There are many types of therapy, but some of the most common are
- Physical therapy: Physical therapists practice a type of rehabilitative health that uses specially designed exercises or equipment to help patients regain or improve their physical abilities. They often focus on the larger muscle groups like the legs or trunk. They may help children learn to walk, sit alone, or do other activities that involve large muscles.
- Occupational therapy: Occupational therapists work with the smaller muscles to help children manipulate tools. For example, they might work on children's hand muscles to facilitate the use of feeding utensils like spoons and writing utensils like crayons.
- Speech therapy: Speech therapists work with the brain functions and the muscles of the mouth and tongue involved in expressive language. While the name reflects the work that they do with speech, they can also help infants and children with feeding and swallowing.

Physical, occupational, and speech therapists are often part of the early intervention or special education teams (for more information, see Chapter 2).

Medical Home

The *medical home* describes care that should be provided in the practice of the pediatrician/primary care provider (PCP). It is a concept that reflects the philosophy of care. The medical home is not a place—it is an approach to providing comprehensive health care in partnership with families. A medical home is composed of pediatricians/PCPs, nurses, and office staff who work together with the patient and family to provide care that is continuous, comprehensive, family-

Benefits of a Medical Home

- Families routinely see the same doctor or other health care professional and office staff who know their child and family.
- The family feels supported at all stages of the child's development.
- Families who have a medical home receive the advice and care they need from their health team in collaboration with other partners as appropriate (eg, caregivers/teachers, social services, early intervention professionals). Families who use a medical home use health care resources appropriately rather than seeking duplicate or wasteful services separately from multiple sources or using emergency departments as their regular source of care better provided in the medical home.
- Caregivers/teachers who participate in the medical home process learn about ways to promote health and help to educate health professionals about quality early childhood education and school programs, sharing typical situations that occur and affect the well-being of their patients in the educational setting. This "mutual education" process helps everyone to decide together what services are available and would be most helpful in meeting the child's and family's needs.
- Caregiver/teacher and health professional discussions about medical homes can lead to identification of community needs and strategies for addressing them. For example, when there are not enough physicians, mental health professionals, or dentists to meet the needs of the population, these 2 professional groups in the community may join to seek strategies to enhance those services. Another example is when caregivers/teachers and health professionals agree that there is a general need for community education about subjects such as the use of smoke detectors, child safety seats, or healthy diet, and start a family educational campaign.
- Because health services are provided in a coordinated way, resources are used efficiently, families are healthier, and money is saved over time.

centered, coordinated, compassionate, culturally effective, and accessible.

The pediatrician/PCP is responsible for coordinating care for the child. Parents should meet with the pediatrician/PCP to create a Care Plan for their child and to share any concerns that arise with the child. Having written observations from school or child care of any concerning signs and symptoms will be very helpful to the pediatrician/PCP. See Chapter 4 for more details.

Pediatric Subspecialists

Many children with chronic medical conditions like diabetes or cystic fibrosis receive much of their medical care from their subspecialty doctor. Other subspecialists may provide occasional consultation but will depend on the child's pediatrician to provide ongoing care for a child. This varies greatly from community to community, so it is important to discuss with parents who should be the primary contact for medical problems.

Glossary of Subspecialists		
Subspecialist	*What They Treat*	*Typical Problems Managed*
Allergist	Allergies	Asthma, anaphylaxis, nasal and skin allergy
Cardiologist	Heart problems	Congenital heart disease, murmurs
Dermatologist	Skin diseases	Eczema
Developmental pediatrician	Developmental delays	Cerebral palsy, attention-deficit/hyperactivity disorder, autism, pervasive developmental disorder, behavioral problems
Ear, nose, and throat surgeon	Ear, nose, and throat	Recurrent ear and throat infections
Endocrinologist	Hormone problems	Diabetes, thyroid disease
Gastroenterologist	Stomach and intestinal problems	Celiac disease, Crohn disease, ulcerative colitis, gastroesophageal reflux disease, liver disease
Geneticist	Inherited diseases	Phenylketonuria, Down syndrome
Hematologist[a]	Blood diseases	Sickle cell, hemophilia, immune thrombocytopenia purpura
Infectious disease	Infectious diseases	HIV, immune problems
Neonatologist	Premature and sick infants	Apnea, follow-up of newborn problems
Nephrologist	Kidney problems	Congenital kidney problems, nephrotic syndrome
Neurologist	Neurologic problems	Seizures, cerebral palsy
Neurosurgeon	Brain and spine problems	Hydrocephalus, spina bifida
Oncologist[a]	Cancer	Leukemia and other cancers
Ophthalmologist	Eye problems	Eye disease of premature newborns, strabismus (crossed eyes)
Pediatric surgeon	General surgery in children	Gastrointestinal surgery, hernias
Pulmonologist	Lung problems	Asthma, cystic fibrosis
Urologist	Urinary system	Urinary reflux, abnormalities of the urinary system

[a]Hematology is often combined with oncology.

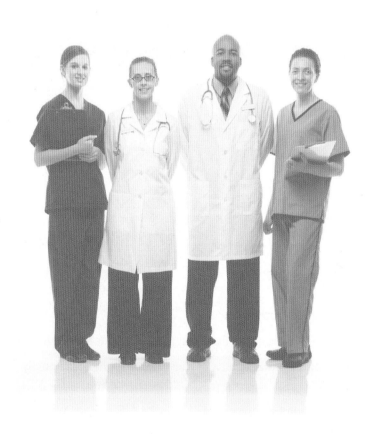

CHAPTER 4

Care Plans

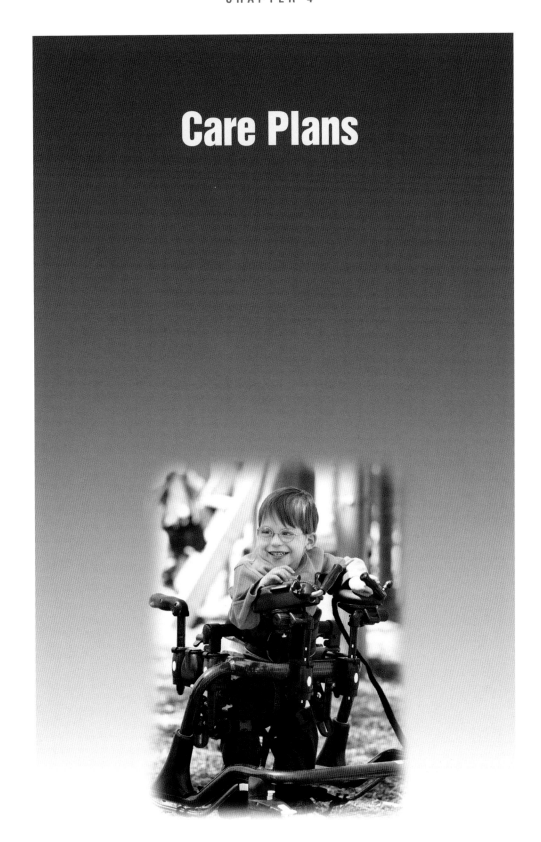

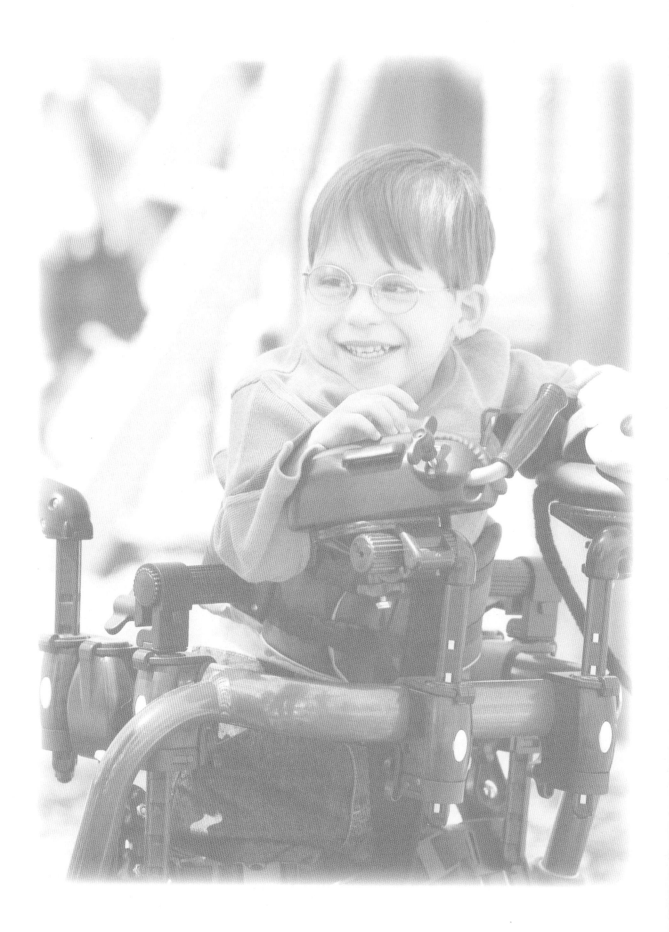

Care Plans

According to a federal study *(National Survey of Children with Special Health Care Needs Chartbook 2005–2006* [US Department of Health and Human Services, 2008]), 14% of children have a special health care need. This special health care need could be anything from asthma to visual impairments. The common theme is that it requires caregivers/teachers to have extra information about the child and to have some plans in place. How do educators get that extra information in a way that can help with planning? This document is called a Care Plan. It may be called by a different name in local areas, but all good Care Plans provide caregivers/teachers with

- Specific medical information
- Special medication or medical procedures that may be required on a routine basis
- Modifications needed in daily activities like diet, transportation, or changes in the physical environment
- Special emergency response information on how to recognize that the child is having a medical emergency and how to respond to the emergency

Care Plans: An Overview

The Care Plan is
- Completed by the child's physician or health care professional
- Reviewed by parents/guardians
- Implemented by caregivers/teachers/school nurses

Caring for Our Children: National Health and Safety Performance Standards: Guidelines for Our-of-Home Child Care Programs, 2nd Edition, states in Standard 8.011d that a plan for the care of ill children shall include, "A procedure to obtain and maintain updated individual emergency care plans for children with special health care needs."

The term *Care Plan* is used by many different groups and it might mean different things to different people (see Table). Herein, the term means a *medical* Care Plan or individual health services plan. There are also plans developed under the Individuals With Disabilities Education Act (IDEA). (Please see Chapter 2 for more details about IDEA.) There are Individualized Education Programs (IEPs) that are developed by the child study team with parents/guardians to outline educational resources that a child might need in school, and there are Individualized Family Service Plans for younger children in the early intervention program who are not yet attending school. These plans may be overseen by a care or service coordinator. Different care managers might be assisting children and their families through managed care organizations, and visiting nurse programs or mental health organizations as well.

If a child with asthma and a severe peanut allergy were enrolling in child care, the Care Plan might include information on the child's asthma medications and whether to give those medicines with a nebulizer (machine) or inhaler (Figure 4-1). It might specify that the child needs to get the medication every day or might only need it for an asthma episode.

The Care Plan should specify what symptoms to watch for. For example, some children only have increased coughing with an asthma episode, some have wheezing which can be heard, and some complain of chest tightness. The Care Plan is a way to capture the individual information about that child and pass the information along to the caregiver/teacher.

Because the child in our example also has a severe allergy to peanuts, it might be necessary to create a peanut-free table at lunch and to make sure that none of the art projects include peanut butter or peanut products. The child might also need

Care Plans		
Type of Care Plan	*Who Creates It*	*Purpose*
Medical Care Plan	Health care professionals	Transmit important health information.
Individualized Family Service Plan	Early intervention team	Outline therapeutic plan for child younger than 3 years with developmental delays.
Individualized Education Program	Special education team in the school district	Outline therapeutic plan for child older than 3 years with educational or developmental needs.
Emergency Care Plan	Health care professionals	A plan for medical emergencies with information about the child for the emergency doctors.

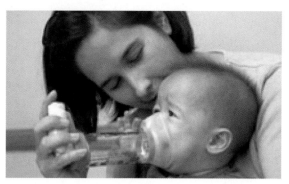

Figure 4-1. Inhaler with spacer for asthma medications.

to avoid outdoor play on high ozone days because of asthma. Chapter 5 has ideas about implementing such modifications.

Emergency planning for this child might include recognizing the signs of a severe allergic reaction and how to administer emergency medications. It would also include the symptoms of a severe asthma episode and what to do.

Which Children Need a Care Plan?

Any child who has extra or special medical needs should have a Care Plan. The child may have chronic medical or special needs on a daily basis, or the child may be at risk for an emergency medical condition. Either way, the Care Plan would explain the symptoms to look for and the care that needs to be given. The Care Plan could be very simple or very complex depending on the child's condition.

Why Do Child Care/Schools Need Care Plans?

- To be informed.
- To develop policies and procedures such as a medication administration policy (see Chapter 6 for more information about giving medication in child care and schools).
- To guide plans for staff education—for example, staff might need to learn about early signs and symptoms of a severe allergic reaction or an asthma episode.
- To plan for administering medications on a routine or an emergent basis.
- To plan for modifications of the diet or environment.
- To plan for emergencies.

What Should a Care Plan Include?

- Diagnosis(es)
- Contact information for family and doctors including subspecialists
- Medication or procedure to be administered
- Allergies
- Dietary modifications
- Activity modifications
- Environmental modifications

- Triggers to avoid
- Symptoms to watch for
- Behavioral modifications
- Emergency response plans
- Suggested special education and skill training for staff

Some Care Plans will be very simple and will not require all these areas to be included. The Quick Reference Sheets in this guide will give you some ideas of what might need to be included if the child has a specific medical problem.

Who Is Responsible for the Care Plan?

Everyone is responsible for the Care Plan! The child's physician or health care professional should complete the Care Plan with input from other health providers and parents. Examples of different types of Care Plans are listed in Chapter 11. Some Care Plans are disease-specific like asthma action plans. Some are geared specifically to emergencies. Some of the most useful Care Plans are generic and allow adaptation for the child's specific medical condition.

Health Care Professional Responsibilities

The health care professional who completes the Care Plan should ensure that the Plan
- Is legible.
- Does not include medical jargon.
- Is complete.
- Is specific for that child.
- Is completed in a timely fashion.

Parent/Guardian Responsibilities

The parent/guardian should
- Have the Care Plan completed in a timely fashion.
- Get updates with changes in the child's medical condition (eg, hospitalizations, change in medications).
- Provide child-specific information (eg, tips for giving medications, signs of impending medical problems).
- Collaborate with the health care professional.
- Review the Care Plan with all those who care for the child.
- Be available when the child has medical problems.
- Facilitate communication between those who care for the child and the health care professional.

Child Care/School Responsibilities

The child care program/school should
- Review the Care Plan.
- Develop an implementation plan (see Chapter 5).
- Meet with parents/guardians to discuss the Care Plan.
- Ensure proper supports are in place for implementing the Care Plan.
- Facilitate any needed staff education and skill training.

The Care Plan is a living document and should be updated frequently, especially after hospitalizations and visits with the doctor.

Tips for Completing the Care Plan

- Have parents/guardians schedule time with the health care professional to complete the form together instead of just dropping it off at the front desk.
- Encourage parents/guardians to prepare before the meeting with their health care professionals by completing the demographic, contact information, and other appropriate sections.
- Parents/guardians should bring details of the medications that the child is taking, especially when a specialist prescribes it and the primary health care professional is completing the form.

Scheduling an actual appointment to complete the Care Plan with the doctor instead of just leaving the form at the office is part of the child's medical care management and is frequently covered by insurance plans. The parent/guardian can give the health care professional information about the structure of the child's educational setting and participate in deciding what is appropriate for the health professional recommendations on the Care Plan. For instance, the doctor might assume that there is a nurse on site or might not realize that the after-school program does not have access to the medications stored in the school nurse's office. Collaboration is critical to creating a good Care Plan.

Care Plans for Schools

Whether the child has an IEP, a Section 504 plan, or neither, the management of special health care needs is the school district's responsibility. Each student with chronic medical conditions and special health care needs should have a written Individual Health Care Plan (IHCP). The school's IHCP is designed to ensure that the child receives the health services he or she needs during the school day (eg, health assessments, treatments, building accommodations, administration of medication). The IHCP represents the physical and mental health guidelines for the individual child. In many, if not most cases, the IHCP is a stand-alone document. That said, these guidelines are extracted and incorporated, as the team determines, into a Section 504 plan or an IEP. One advantage of this is that the plan becomes legally binding and follows the student from one school to another, even state to state.

The IHCP is developed from information provided by the families and the medical home provider and is tailored to the school environment. In addition to the components already described, the IHCP should include provisions for after-school activities, extracurricular activities, and field trips. It

may be similar to the home Care Plan; it may have portions that are codified within the IEP or Section 504 plan. It also includes provisions for self-care in older students. If elements of the IHCP are incorporated in the IEP, care must be taken to notate that minor changes will not necessitate reconvening the entire team unless those changes substantially affect the student's health care and access to educational services.

In the school-aged child, the Care Plan should build in self-efficacy, and the student should contribute to the plan where appropriate. This is especially true at transition times.

Communication among home, the medical home, and the school requires free exchange of protected medical information. Schools are protected by the Family Educational Rights and Privacy Act (FERPA). When health information protected by the Health Insurance Portability and Accountability Act (HIPAA) is accepted by the school, it becomes educational information governed by FERPA, not HIPAA. School staff with a *right to know* (ie, have direct relationship to the student's academic performance) may have access to this information. Schools may create more restrictive access by designating an information gatekeeper (usually the school nurse), who will filter the information so that only the staff determining the child's placement and IEP or Section 504 plan will have access to the entire record.

In districts with school nurses, the Care Plan is generally under their supervision. The National Association of School Nurses (NASN) considers the school nurse to be the case manager for these students in the school setting. In a position paper on the subject, NASN states, "Delivery of health care in the school setting requires the coordination of multiple health and non-health related services. The school nurse has the knowledge, skills, judgment, and critical thinking, inherent in nursing education and authorized through nursing licensure, to perform efficiently in the role as case manager." The Nurse Practice Act is a set of laws that defines the nurse's scope of practice based on the content of the formal education and level of nurse (eg, registered nurse, licensed practical nurse/licensed vocational nurse, nurse practitioner). The scope of practice varies from state to state and can affect school practices such as delegation of procedures and medication. In addition the state Department of Education may set requirements for certification as a school nurse.

Not all school districts have school nurses in every building. According to the Centers for Disease Control and Prevention periodic surveillance of school districts from 2006, 5.8% of states and 19.5% of districts required each school to have at least one full-time school nurse, and 16% of states and 12.2% of districts required a maximum student-to-school nurse ratio. The percentage of schools in which a school nurse participated in the development of IHCPs increased from

59.3% in 2000 to 73.8% in 2006. When a school does not employ a school nurse, the health care coordination should be supervised by one of the following: school district/community physician with child or adolescent health experience, pediatric home care nurse, public health nurse with child and adolescent experience, hospital- or community-based nurse practitioner, or specialist.

To facilitate planning and implementation of appropriate services, training, and education, schools and school districts need to know the extent of chronic medical conditions and special health care needs within their student population.

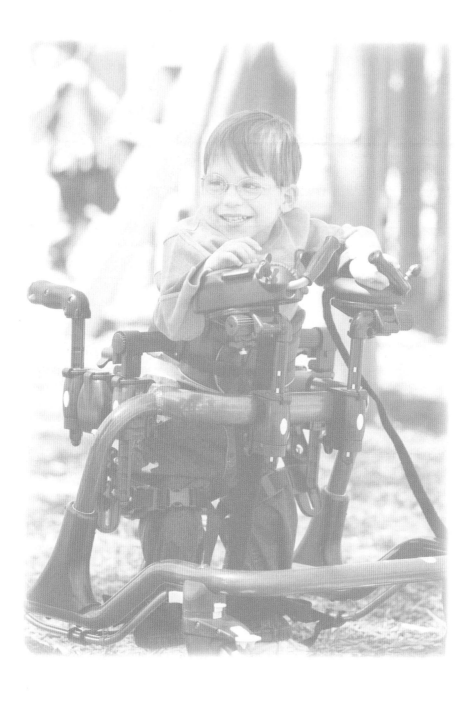

CHAPTER 5

Special Care Plan Implementation Strategies for Caregivers/Teachers

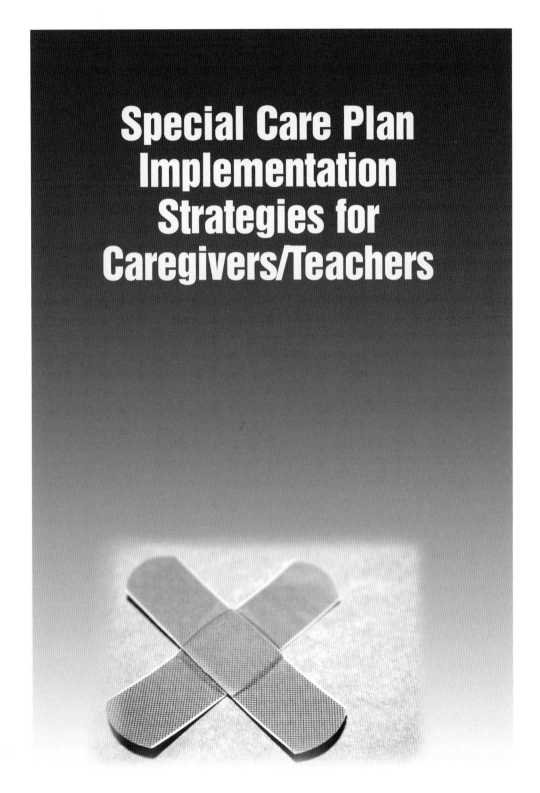

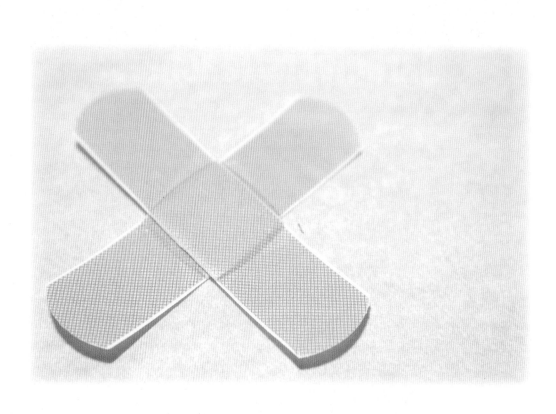

Special Care Plan Implementation Strategies for Caregivers/Teachers

The implementation of a well-developed Special Care Plan for a child in group care or school will vary with every community and family and the complexity of the child's chronic medical condition or special health care needs. This section focuses largely on child care programs, but may also be referred to by states and school districts when reviewing their policies.

Developing and Implementing the Special Care Plan

Parents/guardians should visit the selected program before a child attends to determine what modifications, if any, need to be made and whether any local regulatory agencies need to be consulted to ensure compliance. For example, California Community Care Licensing requires completion of certain forms for conditions such as using inhaled medication or gastric tube feeding.

A tour with the family child care provider, center director, lead teacher, principal, school nurse, or special care coordinator should include the indoor and outdoor areas of the program where children play, sleep, and eat, and also the diapering and toileting, food service, and drop-off and pick-up areas. A parent/guardian can help identify changes in the physical environment that will make for successful inclusion. If there are serious modifications needed such as a ramp or a privacy area for procedures such as catheterization, they need to be defined in writing in a Care Plan. The tour also provides the opportunity for a parent/guardian to observe staff interactions with children and activities that may need to be adapted and included in the plan. For example, for a child with a visual impairment, make certain a barrier-free route is established from areas like the classroom to the toilet room. A brief visit by the child after this tour will introduce the staff and other key personnel to the child and the child to the program.

School personnel/child care center directors or family child care providers also have the opportunity to ask initial questions related to health care needs such as
- How does your child's health care need affect typical activities like playing, eating, sleeping, eliminating, and interacting?
- How and how often is your child affected by the medical condition?
- What are impending signs of trouble and how do we respond?

- Are there other health professionals, such as special education (for children older than 3 years) or early intervention services (for children aged 0–3 years), who are helping you and your child?
- Will they be willing to work with us to help your child, and will you give written consent for us to contact them?
- What, if any, special skills or education will my staff or I need and do you have any ideas who could provide it?
- What medication will your child need while in the program and how is it administered?
- How does the medication affect your child?
- Does your child receive any special treatments and what do we need to know about them?
- Is there any equipment involved and how will it be provided and maintained?
- Who do we contact in case of an emergency?
- Do you have information on the health condition that will help us understand your child's needs?

Answers to these questions will help determine what Care Plan and other forms should be selected from the templates in Chapter 11. The forms will help obtain information from the child's health care professional or other services. A general "Care Plan for Children With Special Health Needs" (page 161) may suffice, or plans for specific conditions such as asthma, allergies, and seizure disorder will provide guidance for specific conditions. Consent forms to share information specific for the care of the child are essential (see samples in Chapter 11), in addition to the usual enrollment forms such as health appraisal, child development, and health history forms.

The next meetings with the parent/guardian should include where appropriate
- The parent/guardian(s).
- The person (eg, special care coordinator, school nurse, director) who serves as the single contact for collecting and coordinating information, training, and overall implementation.
- The lead teacher or primary caregiver(s) who will provide the care and special service.
- The health care professional or consultant, if available, who provides specialized treatment, training, or information.
- The Individualized Education Program (IEP) or Individualized Family Service Plan (IFSP) team if appropriate and required.
- Other caregivers, eg, before- and after-school providers, when possible.

- Ancillary staff such as bus drivers, food service personnel, or janitors may not necessarily be present but should be informed and trained as needed.

At this time, a strategy for implementing the Care Plan can be developed, and needs, goals, and implementation strategies can be defined. The members of the team will vary depending on the nature of the disability. Common health care needs such as food allergies may only require the participation of the parent/guardian, school personnel, and primary caregivers/teachers. More complex needs such as a child with severe developmental and language delay, a gastric feeding tube, and continence challenges will require the input and guidance of several therapists and health care professionals. The child's needs may require the development of an IEP or IFSP (see Chapter 2 and "Questions and Answers: IDEA & Child Care" in Chapter 11). If care is provided in family child care, that provider may be the only caregiver. Parents should be willing to provide consent to share necessary information to those who might be involved in the child's care or to post information where needed to alert those who might be present as volunteers in the program when an emergency related to the child's care occurs.

Deadlines for enrollment of a new child, plus implementation and review dates, can be established. Some child care programs such as Head Start have assessment and review deadlines, generally 30 to 45 days. Lead agencies, such as local school district special education or early intervention programs, have their prescribed review dates, generally every 3 or 6 months. If review dates are not prescribed, the plan should be reviewed or updated anytime there is a change in the health condition or a concern by the educational program, or at least yearly. Training needs, equipment use, and developmental and social needs can be identified. Reports and assessments from various health care professionals, therapists, and education consultants can be compiled, discussed, and integrated, and the need for additional assessments determined. Schedules for visits from outside providers such as a speech or physical therapist, nutritionist, and visiting nurse or physician can be determined.

Staff Development

In addition to standard training for all staff members at orientation, enrollment of a child with chronic medical conditions or special health care needs requires special training to ensure that staff and ancillary personnel (eg, bus driver, food service personnel, janitor, volunteers) have an understanding of the child's special need and ways of working with the child in group care. The training topics are outlined in *Caring for Our Children: National Health and Safety*

Performance Standards: Guidelines for Out-of-Home Child Care Programs, 2nd Edition, Standard 1.024, and include but are not limited to

- Recognizing signs and symptoms of impending medical problems
- Positioning for feeding and handling techniques of children with physical disabilities
- Proper use and care of the individual child's adaptive equipment, including how to recognize defective equipment and to notify parents that repairs are needed
- How different disabilities affect the child's ability to participate in group activities
- Methods of helping the child with special needs to participate in the facility's programs
- Role modeling, peer socialization, and interaction
- Behavior modification techniques, positive rewards for children, promotion of self-esteem, and other techniques for managing difficult behavior
- Grouping of children by skill levels, taking into account the child's age and developmental level
- Intervention for children with special health care conditions
- Communication needs
- Opportunities to discuss similarities and differences with children and staff
- Opportunities for children and staff to explore and ask questions about any equipment or condition

The parent, in collaboration with the primary health care professional, should be involved for typical adaptations. However, even parents who know how to care for their children may not have the skills to teach what they know to others. Confirming the skills and knowledge with the child's primary health care professional is essential. The parents and the child's primary health care professional are most familiar with the child's special needs. Local child care health consultants in the community can be located through the National Child Care Health Consultant Registry (http://hccnsc.edc.org/registry) or the local Child Care Resource & Referral Agency. School nurses can help with training and implementation.

Members of the early intervention team can be especially useful in demonstrating and teaching strategies and treatment procedures. Primary caregivers and ancillary staff should be identified and assigned to receive training. Appropriate staff should have the opportunity to demonstrate their skill in using equipment or other procedures before being left to do it alone. Additional training of staff may be necessary and resources can be obtained from the National Association of Child Care Resource & Referral Agencies (www.naccrra.net) and community-based organizations such as the American Diabetes Association (www.diabetes.org), Food Allergy &

Anaphylaxis Network (www.foodallergy.org), and American Lung Association (www.lungusa.org). See Training Resources on page 200 for further information.

Staff who will be caring for children who require more specialized health procedures such as tube feeding, tracheal suctioning, bladder catheterization, postural drainage, and blood glucose testing should receive on-site training with written directives from the health care professional who prescribed the treatment. A health care professional usually provides the care for the child directly or provides the training in compliance with regulations and state nursing practice acts. The instructions to prepare staff for performing the procedure should include how to prepare for the procedure, how to use and maintain any equipment, and what to do or who to notify in case of complications. The parent/guardian generally provides the equipment and the child's educational program provides enough time to allow for staff training and for staff to perform the procedures once trained. Plans for absence of trained staff should be made.

Model Child Care Policies and School Regulations Support Inclusion

Best practices and policies in a school or child care program
- Promote and protect the health and safety of children and staff.
- Help families understand the program operation.
- Help with regulation and standard compliance.
- Ensure consistent practice.
- Encourage open communication among staff and families.

To be effective, policies should reflect best practices, be developed with multiple inputs, be disseminated and updated routinely, and provide the basis for training.

Basic policies that apply to all child care programs also support inclusion and are well-described in *Caring for Our Children,* 2nd Edition, Standard 8.004 (see Table).

Model Child Care Health Policies; Caring for Our Children, 2nd Edition; *CCHP Health and Safety Checklist;* and sources through the National Resource Center for Health and Safety in Child Care and Early Education provide examples and language for these policies and can be adapted for center or family child care.

Some key resources for states and school districts to refer to when creating and implementing policies addressing students with chronic medical conditions and special health care needs are the American Academy of Pediatrics (AAP) *School Health: Policy & Practice,* 6th Edition, and several AAP policy statements, including
- "Medical Emergencies Occurring at School" (http://aappolicy.aappublications.org/cgi/content/full/pediatrics;122/4/887)
- "Guidelines for the Administration of Medication in School" (http://aappolicy.aappublications.org/cgi/content/full/pediatrics;112/3/697)
- "Disaster Planning for Schools" (http://aappolicy.aappublications.org/cgi/content/full/pediatrics;122/4/895)

Content of Polices		
• Admission and enrollment	• Supervision	• Authorized caregivers
• Safety surveillance	• Discipline	• Health education
• Sanitation and hygiene	• Sleeping	• Evening and night Care Plan
• Child health services	• Medications	• Use of health consultants
• Transportation and field trips	• Emergency plans	• Staff health, training, benefits, and equipment
• Food handling, feeding, and nutrition	• Evacuation plans	• Maintenance of the facility and equipment
• Smoking, prohibited substances, and firearms	• Care of acutely ill children	• Review and revision of policies, plans, and procedures

Communication

A well-developed Care Plan, IFSP, or IEP provides specific information to care for the child, but it is good communication that makes plan implementation work. The informal daily contacts with parents/guardians form the basis of trust essential to make the parent/guardian–caregiver relationship work. Following are some suggestions on communicating with parents/guardians about Care Plans for children with chronic medical conditions and special health care needs:

1. Let the parents/guardians know of the successes and challenges, activities, and special relationships that the child experienced during the day.
2. Provide feedback related to any special services a child may have received.
3. Ask for their ideas for problem solving as you share your concerns and they share theirs.
4. Set up routine conferences allowing parents/guardians and providers to gather their thoughts away from the distraction of the classroom.
5. Take pictures or share the child's work and ask about how other members of the family are doing.
6. Introduce parents/guardians to others families, especially those with similar children and support services; they can be found through the local family resource center, which can be located through the Technical Assistance Alliance for Parent Centers (www.taalliance.org).
7. Avoid mistakes by providing written information describing when medications or procedures were administered and the response to them. This is especially important when there are multiple caregivers or if a before- or an after-school program is involved. Notebooks that are passed along with the child are especially good for sharing information with all parties. Make sure that needed medications and equipment are passed safely and reliably among parents/guardians and caregivers/teachers, or that the medications and equipment are duplicated so all parties can have an adequate supply. For example, most pharmacists are willing to split prescriptions into separate, well-labeled containers.
8. Confidentiality should be maintained at each step in compliance with any laws or regulations that are pertinent to the program such as the Family Educational Rights and Privacy Act (commonly known as FERPA) and Health Insurance Portability and Accountability Act (commonly known as HIPAA).

Children with chronic medical conditions and special health care needs experience a series of transitions during the educational process. These may include, but may not be limited to, transition between early intervention and school, school buildings within a school district, school districts, school and hospital, and school and adulthood, which may include independent living or transfer to another state agency serving adults with disabilities. Each transition represents a challenge for the student, his or her family, and the responsible staff. Schools play an important role in the transitioning. To mitigate these challenges, the family, school, and medical home provider should work together as early as possible to identify special health or safety needs. These needs should be reassessed at least annually and Care Plans and other plans modified accordingly.

Communication with health care professionals can be facilitated by parents/guardians who are engaged in developmental and health screenings and problem solving. Some forms aid communication, such as "Information Exchange on Children With Health Concerns Form" (Chapter 11), which tells a health provider what the child care concern is and provides space for the health care professional to respond to that concern. Parents/guardians and caregivers/teachers must understand that the health care professional or agency cannot reveal personal information without parental/guardian consent. Simple requests for information can often be requested by phone with the parent/guardian or by fax if signed parental/guardian consent is included.

Caring for children with chronic medical conditions and special health care needs may initially seem very demanding and somewhat frightening to caregivers with little experience in caring for these children. However, they should be assured that like parents/guardians, they can learn the adaptations and procedures with good consultation, practice, and supports inherent in a quality educational program.

See Additional Resources (page 197) for more information.

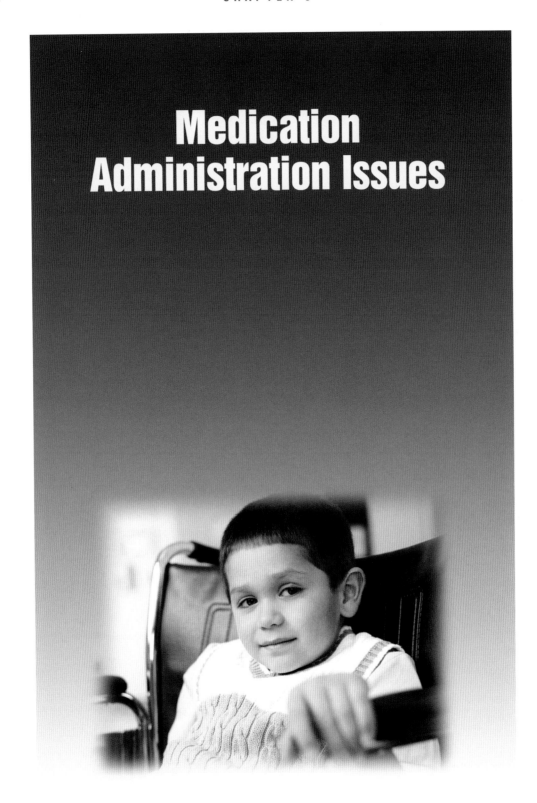

CHAPTER 6

Medication Administration Issues

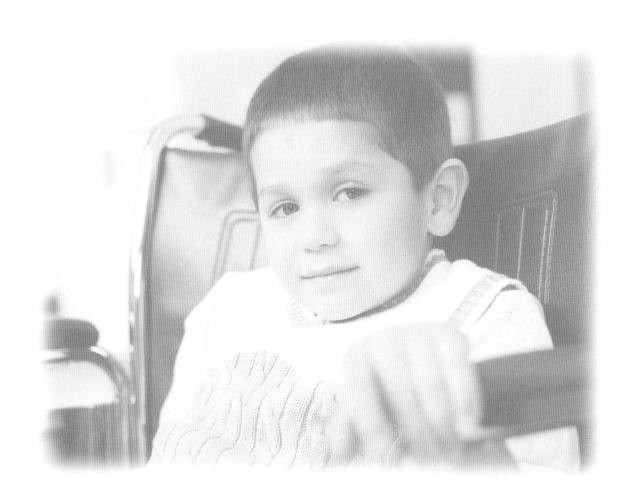

Medication Administration Issues

Children often require medications for short-term illnesses or chronic conditions such as asthma, life-threatening food allergies, or attention-deficit/hyperactivity disorder. In the United States, 14% of children have special health care needs, and 86% of those children require medications daily or when symptoms develop and an immediate response is needed. Although it is preferred that parents/guardians administer medications, all those who care for children for some part of the day need to be prepared and supported to administer medications. Schools and child care facilities may need to provide medications because children in their care need to have medicine in the hours while they are away from home.

Some programs are reluctant to administer medications. In a study in one state, some child care providers reported that they refused to administer medications because they did not have access to or funding to pay for training as well as ongoing health professional guidance. Furthermore, they feared legal action if they made an error. These are understandable concerns that can and should be addressed. Best-practice standards fully support efforts to ensure that caregivers/teachers administer medications safely to children. The Nurse Practice Act, state departments of education, and local boards of health may govern who and how medication is dispensed in schools. Child care regulations and center policy may govern medication administration in child care centers.

Federal Law, Standards, and State Regulations

Caregivers/teachers should be familiar with federal law, state child care and school regulations, and national standards, all of which guide the practice of medication administration in out-of-home settings. According to the Americans With Disabilities Act, schools, child care, and Head Start programs are included under the law and therefore must administer most medications prescribed for children with chronic medical conditions and special health care needs. No program can screen out a child because of a disability or refuse to make a reasonable accommodation such as administering a required medication. In fact, schools and child care programs are at greater risk for legal action if they refuse to admit or accommodate a child with a chronic medical condition or special health care need who requires medication (see "Americans With Disabilities Act: Commonly Asked Questions Related to Giving Medicine in Child Care" in Chapter 11).

Caring for Our Children: National Health and Safety Performance Standards: Guidelines for Out-of-Home Child Care Programs, 2nd Edition, includes 34 standards on safe medication administration practices in child care settings.

National Association for the Education of Young Children accreditation and Head Start Performance Standards include specific criteria to ensure safe medication administration practices. *School Health: Policy & Practice,* 6th Edition, notes that American Academy of Pediatrics (AAP) and National Association of School Nurses statements "recommend that the administration of all medications in schools meet specific guidelines that include compliance with the state's nurse practice act and other applicable laws and policies." All of these guidelines emphasize the importance of a comprehensive medication administration training program for caregivers/teachers conducted by a licensed health professional, with parent permission and prescriber authorization.

State child care regulations vary widely. For example, as of 2005,
- One state had no regulations on medication administration.
- Forty-eight states required parent permission for medication administration.
- Forty five mandated written instructions.
- Forty four required that providers maintain records of medication administration.
- Only 8 states included medication administration training for child care providers as a regulatory requirement.

School personnel and child care providers should be aware of their state regulations addressing medication administration but should adhere to best-practice standards to ensure safety and reduce errors. States and school districts can refer to the AAP policy statement, "Guidelines for the Administration of Medication in School" (http://aappolicy.aappublications.org/cgi/content/full/pediatrics;112/3/697), for guidance in developing state and local policies.

Nursing Delegation and Medication Administration

Administering medications is a component of nursing practice. In states where state regulations do not authorize personnel who are neither family members nor licensed health professionals to administer medications, caregivers/teachers do not have legal authority to administer medications. They are, in effect, "practicing nursing without a license." Many state boards of nursing have addressed this issue by working with child care licensing agencies and school health regulatory bodies. Furthermore, nursing boards often act in collaboration with schools and child care agencies to promote high standards of medication administration and increase children's health and safety. Because some state licensing agencies follow the rules set forth by state nurse practice acts, check specific state requirements.

Best-Practice Medication Administration: Essential Elements

Best-practice medication administration in children's programs should include the following key elements:

Preparing to Administer Medication

Medication Administration Policy

A medication administration policy should include a statement of intent, procedures and practices, application (specifically, whom the policy applies to), communication (how and to whom the policy will be shared), references, and review including effective date and renewal date.

Policy should include how medications will be labeled, stored, and disposed of, as well as documenting medication administration and side effects.

Prescriber Authorization

To ensure correct dosing, caregivers/teachers should request detailed written authorizations and instructions for all medications, including over-the-counter (OTC) medications such as acetaminophen (Tylenol is one brand of acetaminophen) and cough and cold medications (if recommended). If program personnel are uncertain about instructions, they should inform parents that they need authorization to speak to the prescriber or pharmacist before administering medications.

Parent Permission

Parents should complete a written authorization granting the child's program permission to administer all prescription and OTC medications. Parents should also administer the first dose of medication at home in the event that there is an unexpected reaction with the first dose.

Medication Administration Log

Programs should keep a medication administration record (MAR) for each child and each medication ordered. The MAR should include
- Child's name
- Address
- Date of birth
- Name of medication
- Dosage ordered and method of administration
- Pharmacy and phone number
- Name of authorized prescriber

- Date, time, and dosage at each administration
- Food and medication allergies
- Date medication is started and ended
- Signature of provider administering the medication
- Side effects
- Adverse reactions
- Errors
- Level of cooperation of the child
- If unused medication was returned to the parent

Programs should maintain a copy of this record for several years. Length of time is determined by the regulations of the oversight state agency or other applicable legal requirements. If in doubt, consult an attorney.

See Chapter 11 for sample medication administration policies and forms.

Training

All personnel who plan to administer medications should complete a training conducted by a licensed health professional who is knowledgeable about medication administration, such as a nurse, physician, physician assistant, or pharmacist. While parents can provide helpful strategies in administering medications to their child, they may inadvertently give incorrect information, such as incorrect dose and frequency of administration. Regardless, caregivers/teachers are ultimately responsible for administering these medications, and if given incorrectly, the caregiver/teacher is at fault, not the parent. Therefore, training by a health professional is essential and should include

Reading Medication Labels

Labels should include date, name of child, prescriber and pharmacy including phone number, name of medication, dose, directions, amount of medication in the container, and expiration date. Knowledge of the exact amount of medication is especially important for controlled substances, such as methylphenidate (Ritalin and Concerta are brand-name examples), to monitor appropriate use. Controlled substances, a group of drugs with potential for addiction and illegal use, are subject to specific federal and state laws.

Principles and Techniques for Medication Administration

Caregivers/teachers should be taught various routes, such as oral (eg, liquids, tablets, caplets, capsules), topical (eg, creams, ointments, drops), inhalant (eg, nebulizer, metered dose inhaler, sprays), and automatic injectables (EpiPen and Twinject are examples of epinephrine injections). Program personnel without health professional licenses may not be able to administer medications by some of these routes; state regulations may specify. For example, some states allow administration of medications rectally and via injection or an automated delivery system such as an insulin pump. Other states only allow these routes with a special waiver and demonstration of competence after training by a health professional. Children of various ages including infants, toddlers, preschool, and school-age have different issues with how they take medications; this should be covered in the training.

Side Effects, Adverse Reactions, and Allergic Reactions

When educational programs accept medications, they are responsible for observing for

1. Side effects, such as sleepiness.
2. Adverse reactions (ie, an unexpected or potentially dangerous reaction such as vomiting).
3. Allergic reactions, which might be mild (ie, a rash) or life threatening (ie, difficulty breathing). If a serious adverse reaction or an allergic reaction occurs, emergency medical services should be called immediately.

Information about drug side effects and adverse reactions is available through pharmacies. Program personnel should ask families for information about drug side effects and adverse reactions when parents ask that the program staff administer medication.

Safe Handling, Storage, and Disposal of Medications

Medications should be locked in a cabinet or container and out of the reach of children. If refrigeration is required, the medication should be in a secure container in the refrigerator. Controlled substances, such as methylphenidate (Ritalin is one brand name), may require additional monitoring and storage requirements. In general, program personnel should keep careful count of these drugs on the MAR and a witness, if available, should cosign administration. Emergency medications, such as epinephrine injections (EpiPen is one brand name) for life-threatening allergies and diazepam rectal (Diastat) for seizures, should be easily accessible but out of the reach of children. Emergency medications should always be available indoors, outdoors, or on a field trip. If parents do not remove unused medications from the program, the program staff should contact a pharmacy for instructions as to how to properly dispose of medications. Controlled substances usually require special precautions.

Precautions to Avoid Errors and Actions in the Event of an Error

1. A space should be well lit, clean, and reserved for preparing medications so that the staff involved in medication administration are not distracted and are less likely to make an error. Supplies should be organized and easily accessible.

2. Staff should be familiar with the child receiving medication. The person who prepares the medication should administer the medication. Review the MAR before administering a medication and document immediately after administration.
3. The 5 rights of medication administration should be ensured at 3 stages of the process—when the medication is taken out of storage, immediately before administering to the child, and after administering the medication.
   - Right child
   - Right medication
   - Right dose
   - Right route
   - Right time

Errors include wrong child, medication, dose, route, and time (or omitting the dose), and giving the medication without permission to administer it. In a school or child care center, if a medication error occurs, the supervising staff person (eg, principal, head teacher, director) should be notified, and parents should be contacted. If the child is demonstrating serious symptoms, such as difficulty breathing or change of consciousness, emergency medical services/911 should be called first. Errors should be recorded on a Medication Incident Report (see page 149). Staff should contact the prescriber or poison control for more information, as well as the parents.

Standard Precautions

Standard precautions mean taking precautions, such as hand washing when administering medications. Gloves are necessary only when there is a potential risk of exposure to blood. Providers should always wash their hands before and after administering medications. Similarly, children should wash their hands if they handle medications.

Demonstration, Return Demonstration, and Written Posttest

Training should include demonstration of proper techniques and return demonstration by the participants—the instructor should show the trainees the technique, and the trainee should demonstrate the technique for the instructor. In addition, a written posttest of the information included in the course helps to ensure that the staff understands the rationale for the procedures that have been taught, demonstrated, and return demonstrated. This component of the training helps the recipients retain their competence. Also, the written posttest is an opportunity to test literacy skills that are essential for interpreting medication orders, drug labels, and drug information.

Individualized Health Care Plan

All children should have a health assessment prior to enrollment, but children with chronic medical conditions and special health care needs require additional information in a Care

Plan. (See Chapter 4 for more information.) Some medications, such as an epinephrine injection (EpiPen) and insulin, require explicit instructions for each child. In that circumstance, program personnel should have not only the prescriber and parent authorizations, but also a completed Care Plan. This can be part of the Care Plan or a separate document. The prescriber should complete the plan so that the program personnel have clear instructions. Every child who will get medication, even OTC medications, needs an individualized Care Plan, but children with chronic medical conditions and special health care needs require a more detailed plan.

Communication With Parents

It is essential that parents and program staff communicate orally and in writing about all medications that are administered in the program, whether these medications are administered daily or on an as-needed basis. Similarly, parents should always inform program staff if children were given medications during the evening or morning before attending the program.

Ongoing Support by a Health Consultant

Health consultants, especially nurses, physicians, and physician assistants, can support programs by providing medication administration training and periodic review of medication administration practices and policies. This is especially important when there is no licensed health professional such as a school nurse on staff.

Advocating for Training and Support

Administering medications to children is an important and serious responsibility for program staff. Therefore, they deserve support, especially access to comprehensive medication administration training programs by licensed health professionals and ongoing support from a health professional who serves as a health consultant. Many states have developed training programs and provide access to health consultants to ensure safe medication administration practices (see Additional Resources on pages 200 and 201). In those states where programs are not developed, program staff may contact health professionals through state chapters of organizations, such as the AAP, National Association of Pediatric Nurse Practitioners, and American Nurses Association, to seek assistance.

See Additional Resources (page 197) for more information.

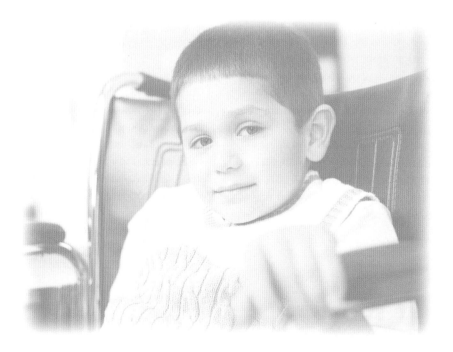

Handling Symptoms That Develop While a Child Is in Child Care or School

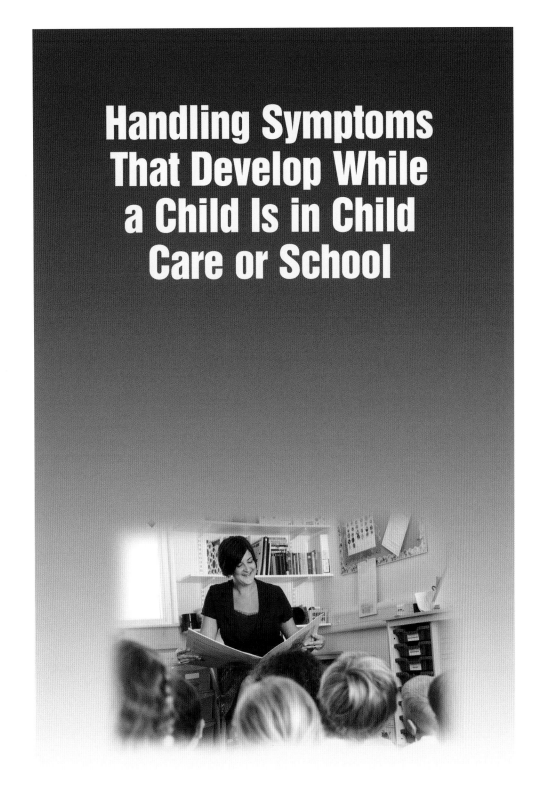

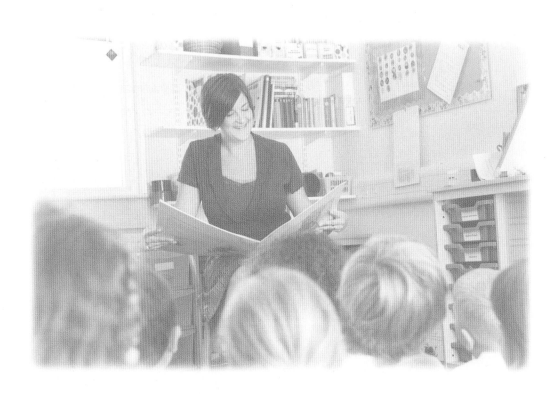

Handling Symptoms That Develop While a Child Is in Child Care or School

Many children will develop medical conditions while in the care of people other than their parents/guardians. Caregivers/teachers may be the first people to notice certain symptoms, especially because they have more opportunities than most parents to observe and compare individual children with a group of same-age children. It's easier to define *normal* and spot unusual behaviors or attributes when you have experience with caring for a number of healthy children around the same age. Also, the pressures of daily routines for many parents may limit their observations of their children. They must focus on dressing and feeding their children and themselves to get out the door in the morning and to get to bed at the end of the day. In addition to lacking a frame of reference to compare their child with other children and feeling rushed and tired, some parents do tag-team parenting and have little time to share observations with the other parent.

While it is not wise for people without medical professional training to start diagnosing children with medical problems, it is wise to call attention to troublesome symptoms such as a child who is losing weight or is unable to participate in physical activities. Caregivers/teachers are often the first to notice developmental delays or problems with vision or hearing. They may notice what a child eats and may discover abnormalities in urine or stool. It is important to share concerns about these observations with parents/guardians.

Parents/guardians want what is best for their children, but they are not always eager to hear about problems or concerns. In addition to providing an in-person discussion, it is helpful to put concerns in writing so parents can review them as convenient and share them with the child's health care professional. The description of the concerns should be as objective as possible, describing observations without suggesting a diagnosis or cause. Be specific about the time and frequency of the symptoms. Ask parents/guardians what they have observed and what they think about the observations being made in the program. Plan with parents/guardians for follow-up to be sure something is done as a next step to determine whether there is a problem that needs special care.

Another tool that may be helpful is the "Information Exchange on Children With Health Concerns Form" in Chapter 11 on page 153. This form helps organize observations, and the parent/guardian can bring the paper to the child's health care professional. The form can be returned by the health care professional with a response if the parents consent. This form can be used for infectious diseases as well as other concerns.

Hints for Recording Observations

- Be objective.
- Be specific.
- Note the time of day that the symptom occurs and what the child is doing.
- Note the frequency and severity of the symptom.
- Observations such as, "Johnny has a dry cough that occurs more during nap time," are more helpful than, "Johnny coughs a lot."

Important Symptoms to Note

- Chronic cough associated with difficulty breathing
- Difficulty breathing without cough
- Wheezing
- Excessive tiredness without known illness
- Stool pattern (eg, chronic diarrhea, blood in stool, constipation)
- Urine pattern (eg, more frequent urination, blood in urine, foul smell to urine)
- Weight loss
- Pain (Note frequency, severity, and location.)
- Inattentiveness (Is it inability to see or hear? Is it a staring spell where the child does not seem to "be there"?)
- Does not seem to see well
- Does not seem to hear well
- Not meeting normal developmental milestones
- Chronic vomiting without known illness
- Scratching or complaints of itching

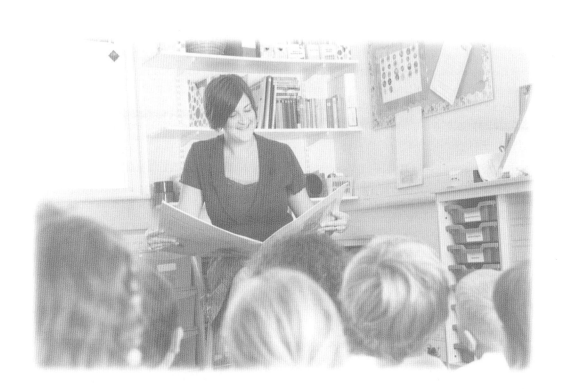

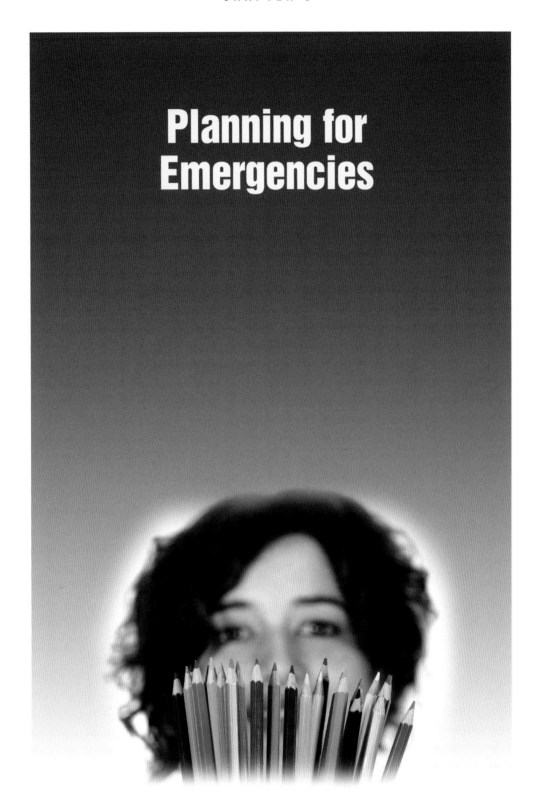

CHAPTER 8

Planning for Emergencies

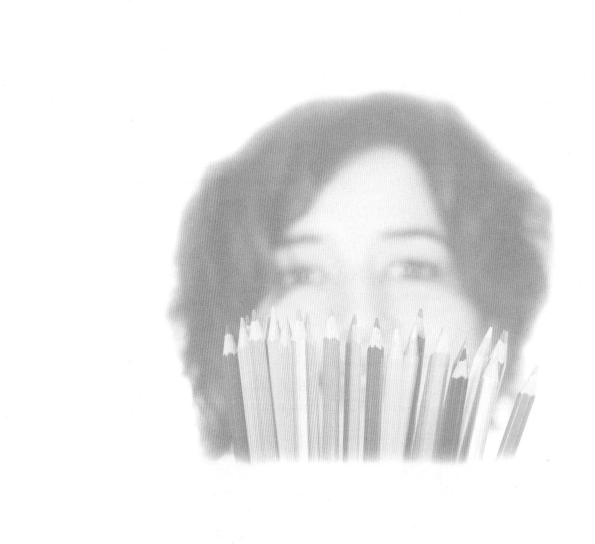

Planning for Emergencies

Not all emergencies are equal. There can be more than one type of emergency.
- Individual/child emergencies, such as a seizure or an allergic reaction—preparation for these types of emergencies are addressed in the Quick Reference Sheets in Chapter 10.
- Programmatic emergency, such as a fire or weather-related emergency—planning for these types of emergencies should be done together with local emergency response teams.

Some universal issues apply when planning for individual emergencies.
- Is there a Care Plan in place with emergency information?
- Who will care for the child and do the required first aid?
- Who will call emergency medical services/911?
- Who will contact parents/guardians?
- Who will care for the other children and clear the area?
- What staff training needs to occur on recognizing the symptoms of an impending or actual emergency? Which staff members need that training?
- What medications or files need to be brought with the child?

The medical Care Plan should address potential individual child emergencies. The Care Plan should be updated frequently, especially after
- Hospitalizations
- Major procedures
- Significant illnesses
- Changes in medications

Programmatic emergencies also require planning. The chronic medical conditions and special needs of certain children need to be worked into the general emergency plans for the program. Some questions to include are
- Who will take the children's medications when a building is evacuated?
- Will any children need special assistance with evacuation?
- Will special supplies be needed for a prolonged emergency?
- Is there need for emergency power for any essential specialized equipment? What equipment is essential or optional?

Who needs to be involved in emergency planning?
- Parents/guardians
- Caregivers and directors
- Health care professionals to complete the Care Plan

Emergency planning should be a collaborative effort.

When to Call Emergency Medical Services (and Also Notify Parents)

Call emergency medical services (EMS)/911 immediately for any of the following:
- Anytime you believe a child needs immediate medical assessment and treatment that cannot wait for parents to take the child for care.
- Fever in association with abnormal appearance, difficulty breathing, or a problem with circulation indicated by an abnormal skin color, such as looking exceptionally pale, having a bluish skin tone, or having skin that is exceptionally pink.
- Multiple children affected by injury or serious illness at the same time.
- A child is acting strangely, is much less alert, or is much more withdrawn than usual.
- Difficulty breathing or unable to speak.
- Skin or lips that look blue, purple, or gray.
- Rhythmic jerking of arms and legs and a loss of responsiveness (seizure—except for a child who is known to have seizures and for whom a Care Plan is in place for management of seizures without calling EMS/911).
- Unresponsive.
- Decreasing responsiveness.
- After a head injury, decreasing level of alertness, confusion, headache, vomiting, irritability, or difficulty walking.
- Vomiting blood.
- Severe stiff neck (limiting child's ability to put chin to chest) with headache and fever.
- Severe dehydration with sunken eyes, lethargy, no tears, and not urinating.
- Suddenly spreading purple or red rash.
- A large volume of blood in the stools.
- Hot- or cold-weather injuries (eg, frostbite, heat exhaustion).

Situations That Require Urgent Medical Attention

These conditions do not necessarily need emergency medical services/911 or ambulance transport if parent notification and transport to medical care can be achieved within an hour or so.

- Fever in a child of any age who looks more than mildly ill
- Elevated temperature for a child who is younger than 2 months (60 days), with an axillary (armpit) temperature of more than 100.5°F (38.1°C) or 101°F (38.3°C) rectally
- Appearing and acting very ill for a child of any age
- Severe vomiting or diarrhea
- An injury that may require medical treatment, such as a cut that does not hold together after it is cleaned
- Any animal bite that breaks the skin
- Venomous bites or stings with spreading local redness and swelling, or evidence of general illness
- Any medical condition that is outlined in the child's Care Plan as requiring medical attention

Do-Not-Resuscitate Plans in Schools

The percentage of schools in which health services staff were required to follow do-not-resuscitate (DNR) orders increased from 29.7% in 2000 to 46.2% in 2006. It is essential for school systems to be prepared to address requests from families and their physicians about DNR orders (see "Elements of a Do-Not-Resuscitate Plan for Schools" in Chapter 11). Schools should be aware of any legalities or policies in their individual state.

See Additional Resources (page 197) for more information.

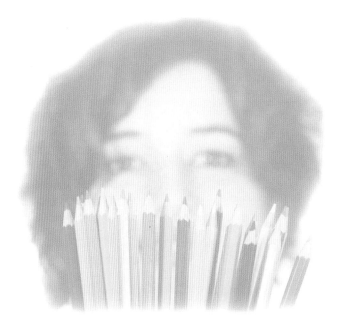

How to Use the Quick Reference Sheets

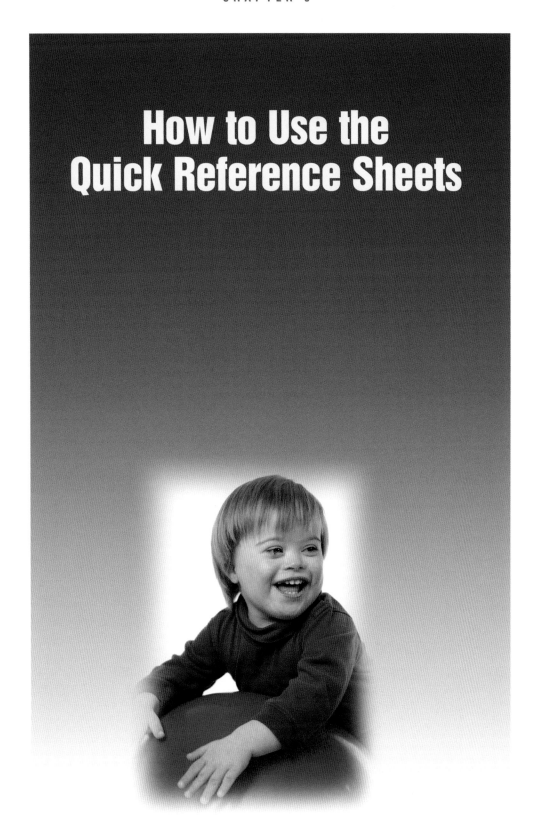

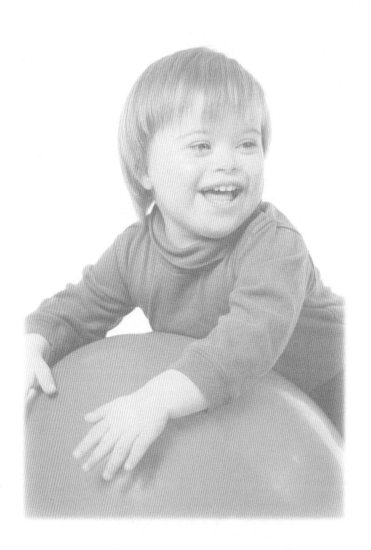

How to Use the Quick Reference Sheets

Each Quick Reference Sheet (QRS) is intended to provide information about a specific condition and some of the problems that might be faced by children with the condition. Remember that not all children with the condition will have *all* the problems mentioned in the QRSs. The structure of the QRSs is as follows (not all conditions will include all categories):

• **What is the condition?** This section provides a brief overview of the medical condition. The resources listed at the end of each QRS provide options for more information.

• **How common is it?**

• **What are some characteristics of children with the condition?** This section gives an idea of some common characteristics of children with this condition and an overview of areas that might be challenging.

• **Who is the treatment team?** This is an overview of some of the health professionals who may be involved in the care of this condition.

• **What are some elements of a Care Plan for this condition?** Guidance on specialized Care Plans for specific conditions is provided here.

• **What adaptations may be needed?** Some adaptations that might be helpful are covered, including medications, dietary considerations, physical environmental, and transportation considerations.

  ~ **Medications.** Please review Chapter 6, "Medication Administration Issues," and see Chapter 11 for forms that might be helpful in medication administration. The most typical types of medications for each condition will be covered. Many children do not require these medications at all, and many children will receive all their medications at home. It is important to know what types of medications a child is taking even if the child does not need to have them administered by program staff, in case a side effect or an allergic reaction occurs while the child is away from home. Preventive vaccinations, though not technically medications, are also covered in this section when applicable.

  ~ **Dietary considerations**. Many children with chronic medical conditions and special health care needs will require a special diet. Sometimes this will be very strict; other times there might just be suggested guidelines. It is important to know the difference.

  ~ **Physical environment.** This includes

    ❖ **Special equipment.** This section will cover the types of equipment that the child might use. Some of this equipment will be essential to the child's well-being; some might be optional. Some types of equipment might be used only in an emergency.

    ❖ **Accommodations.** This will give ideas of how to change the physical environment or adapt the daily schedule to best take care of the child. Adaptations might include spending individual time with the child or changing certain types of play.

  ~ **Transportation considerations.** Here are special instructions for when a child is being transported (eg, to and from child care/school, on a field trip).

• **What should be considered an emergency?** This will cover the types of individual emergencies that the child might experience, such as a seizure, or any planning that might need to take place for a programmatic emergency like a fire. Please see Chapter 8 for further details.

• **What types of training or policies are advised?** This section will suggest special training that staff will require or policies that should be in place.

• **What are some related Quick Reference Sheets?** Other QRSs within the guide may contain pertinent information. This section is particularly important in QRSs that function as overviews of large topics (ie, allergies, altered immunity, bleeding disorders, heart conditions, and premature newborns [preemies]).

• **What are some resources?** This is a quick reference guide and therefore limited in the amount of information that can be provided about a particular condition. There are multiple resources and Web sites that have great information that should be explored. Look for trusted information produced by government agencies, children's hospitals, or well-recognized organizations. Try to look for information that is specific to children because adult medical conditions can be very different. Listing of resources within this book does not imply endorsement by the American Academy of Pediatrics.

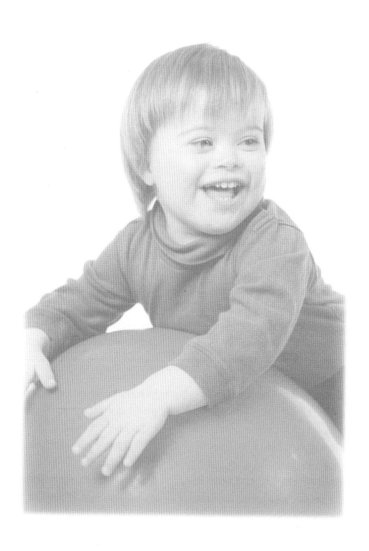

CHAPTER 10

Quick Reference Sheets

No permission is necessary to make single copies for noncommercial, educational purposes.

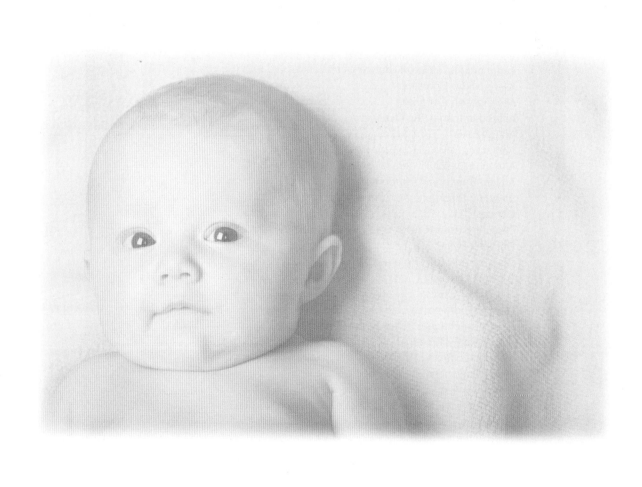

Achondroplasia (Short Stature Conditions)

What is achondroplasia (short stature conditions)?

- More than 100 specific conditions have been identified that can cause short stature. Some of these involve a genetic bone disorder in which the bones do not grow and develop normally.
- Achondroplasia is the most common short stature condition. Children affected with achondroplasia have very short arms and legs while their torso is normal size. Their heads are often large.

How common is it?

- Achondroplasia occurs in all races and with equal frequency in males and females, and affects about 1 in every 26,000 children.
- There are an estimated 10,000 individuals with achondroplasia in the United States.

What are some characteristics of children with achondroplasia?

- Features or effects of achondroplasia include
  - ~ Short arms and legs
  - ~ A large head with a prominent forehead
  - ~ Small midface with a flattened nasal bridge
  - ~ Spinal curvature; back and neck problems
  - ~ Short fingers and toes; extra space between middle and ring fingers
  - ~ Crowded or crooked teeth
  - ~ Bowleg (varus) or knock-knee (valgus) deformities
  - ~ Frequent ear infections
  - ~ Vision problems
  - ~ Hearing loss
  - ~ Respiratory and breathing problems
  - ~ Extra fluid within the brain (hydrocephalus)
  - ~ Normal intelligence
- Overall, development is usually normal, yet children with achondroplasia may reach motor milestones of development slowly.
  - ~ For instance, good head control may not occur until the infant is 7 or 8 months old, because it takes longer to develop the muscular strength necessary to control the large head.
  - ~ Though there are exceptions, many of these children do not walk until relatively late, often between 24 and 36 months.

- Weight control is a frequent and lifelong problem for many people with this disorder. Children and adults must be careful of their nutrition because they tend to gain weight easily.

Who is the treatment team?

- Children with achondroplasia will often see pediatric specialists in dentistry, orthopedics (bone), and otolaryngology (ear, nose, and throat) for their complications.
- Physical and occupational therapy may be needed to help these children achieve normal motor milestones.
- Sometimes surgery is done to help with some of the related physical problems.
- Children who are younger than 3 years may receive therapies through *early intervention* services.
- For children 3 years and older, *special education and related services* are available through public schools to provide the accommodations necessary for school achievement and adaptation.

What adaptations may be needed?

Physical environment

Care Plans may include
- Adaptive equipment to support the head and spine of these children when they are younger.
- As they grow, physical adaptations (eg, lowered doorknobs, blackboards, foot supports for desks and toilets) can be used for many activities of daily living to promote independence.
- Many children will appear younger than their age because of their short stature. Be sure to take their age and normal intelligence into account as you interact with them.
- Many children are at risk for teasing because of their physical appearance. Work to foster self-confidence with the child as well as understanding among his classmates.
- When conducting physical activity in class, be aware that jumping can cause unnecessary stress on joints, especially the spine. Low-impact activity is encouraged.
- Gymnastics and contact sports should be avoided because of potential risk of spine injury. Swimming and biking are encouraged. Adaptive foot pedals on bicycles to accommodate short limbs are helpful.
- Be aware of possible hearing loss in a child who does not respond to you.

➤continued

Achondroplasia (Short Stature Conditions), continued

What should be considered an emergency?

Notify parents/guardians immediately for
- Unexplained numbness or tingling in the arms and legs
- Change in gait when walking
- Change in bowel or bladder control

What are some resources?

- Little People of America, www.lpaonline.org
- Human Growth Foundation, www.hgfound.org, 800/451-6434

American Academy
of Pediatrics

DEDICATED TO THE HEALTH OF ALL CHILDREN™

Allergic Skin Conditions

What are allergic skin conditions?

- There are different types of allergic skin conditions.
  - ~ Eczema (atopic dermatitis) is a long-lasting skin condition in which the skin is overly sensitive to many things. It can affect older children most often in the inside of the elbows, back of the knees, wrists, and neck. In younger children, it may just cause dry, rough patches of skin, particularly in the face and trunk. Sometimes the patches become open or even infected. It may appear thickened and leathery and occasionally leave scars.
  - ~ Hives (urticaria) are patches of itchy, swollen skin that move to various parts of the body. They can be small and look like insect bites, or the patches can blend together to form bigger areas. Hives are always very itchy and are sometimes made worse by pressure, heat, or stress. Hives do not scar or leave marks; however, scratching the hives can lead to a secondary infection, which may require further treatment.
  - ~ Contact dermatitis is caused by a reaction to something touching the skin. Two common examples are poison ivy and a rash around the belly button in people who are allergic to nickel (which is often found in fasteners on waistbands of pants). It may occur in the diaper area if the baby is allergic to the scent or dye used in the diaper. Contact dermatitis usually goes away when the irritant is removed.
- None of these conditions are contagious.

How common are they?

Estimates are that up to 20% of infants and young children may be affected by eczema at some point. There is no good data about how frequently hives and contact dermatitis occur.

What are some characteristics of children with allergic skin conditions?

- Children with eczema tend to have allergies and may have other signs of hay fever such as nasal congestion, sneezing, or itchy eyes. Children with hives or contact dermatitis do not always have other allergy symptoms.
- Food allergies, nasal allergies (allergic rhinitis), and asthma are more common in children with eczema.
- Eczema can be mild or severe.
- Eczema and hives may come and go especially in allergy season, but are commonly present all year long.

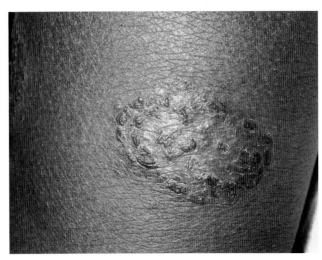
Child with an oval crusted eczema lesion

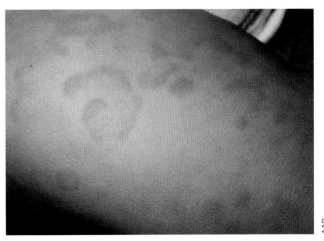
Child with urticaria wheals with multiple shapes

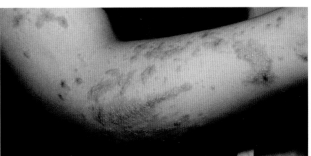
Child with contact dermatitis

➤continued

Allergic Skin Conditions, continued

- Children may scratch their skin and cause a skin infection, and they can be irritable if they are itchy.
- Eczema can be a lifelong condition but tends to have periods where it is better and worse. It often improves by school age.
- Hives can occur periodically but tend to resolve within a week or two.

Who is the treatment team?

- The primary care provider in the medical home
- Allergists and dermatologists

What adaptations may be needed?

Medications

- Medications can be given to relieve the symptoms or cure the condition. Some of these medications are prescription and others are over the counter.
- Moisturizers.
- Antihistamines.
  - ~ Classic—diphenhydramine (Benadryl), hydroxyzine (Atarax), and others. These medications can cause drowsiness in some children. Oddly enough, some children become hyperactive with these medications and it is often difficult to predict what the reaction will be beforehand in each child.
  - ~ Non-drowsy—cetirizine (Zyrtec), loratadine (Claritin), and fexofenadine (Allegra). These medications tend to cause less drowsiness but may not control the itch as well.
- Steroids can be applied as a cream or an ointment. They can also be given orally in severe cases. There can be skin changes if strong steroid creams are used for prolonged periods. Side effects of oral steroids include appetite and mood changes, especially if used for more than a few days.
- Immune modulators like tacrolimus (Protopic) or pimecrolimus (Elidel) are sometimes used in eczema.
- Injected epinephrine (EpiPen) may be prescribed if the child has more serious associated allergies (anaphylaxis).
- Antibiotics are used if a bacterial skin infection is making the eczema worse.
- Caregivers should be given information about any medications the children are taking.

Dietary considerations

Avoid food allergens.

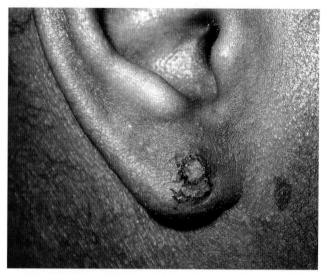

Child with contact dermatitis from the nickel in an earring

Physical environment

- Children may need to avoid things that aggravate their allergy like latex, food, creams, metals, or perfumes.
- Extremes of temperature can aggravate some skin conditions but has to be balanced with the child's need to play. Avoid dust, perfumes, chemicals, and furry animals. Avoid wetting and drying the skin. Special precautions may be necessary for swim activities.
- Eczema is helped by frequent moisturizing of the skin. You may want the child to decorate a pot to put the moisturizing cream in.
- Avoid contact with other blistering skin conditions like a cold sore or chickenpox.
- Try to relieve itching with cool compresses.
- Avoid tight-fitting or scratchy clothing like wool. Sand or dust may make itching worse.
- Avoid vigorous rubbing of the child's skin when drying after cleaning.
- It can be frustrating for children to hear "Don't scratch!" all day, so try distraction—read a story or do a special activity.

What should be considered an emergency?

- Acute hives can be a sign of anaphylaxis, or they can just be a skin problem. Be very aware of other symptoms such as breathing difficulty, throat swelling, color changes, or stomach cramps in a child who has hives. Call emergency medical services/911 if these or any other serious symptoms develop.

➤continued

Allergic Skin Conditions, continued

- If the child has injectable epinephrine prescribed, use it as directed.
- Eczema and contact dermatitis are not emergencies.

What types of training or policies are advised?

- Avoiding triggers
- First aid for rashes

What are some resources?

- National Institute of Arthritis and Musculoskeletal and Skin Diseases (part of the National Institutes of Health), www.niams.nih.gov
- American Academy of Dermatology, www.aad.org
- National Eczema Society, www.eczema.org

American Academy
of Pediatrics

DEDICATED TO THE HEALTH OF ALL CHILDREN™

Allergies: An Overview

What are allergies?

- *Allergy* is the term that is used to describe the body's over-reaction to something that it views as foreign or different.
- The body reacts by releasing histamine and other substances that cause allergic symptoms.
- There are many different types of allergic reactions; some are minor and annoying, but some are serious and life threatening.
- One form of a serious allergic reaction is called anaphylaxis (see Anaphylaxis on page 61).
- Some other examples of allergic reactions are
  ~ Stuffy nose
  ~ Runny nose
  ~ Itchy, watery eyes
  ~ Hives (urticaria)
  ~ Eczema (atopic dermatitis)
  ~ Contact dermatitis
  ~ Wheezing
  ~ Itching of roof of mouth
  ~ Swelling of throat or mouth
  ~ Swelling of the skin (angioedema)
  ~ Stomach cramps
- A child can be allergic to many things. Some children have a tendency toward allergies and may have many of the symptoms. The things that people are allergic to are called *allergens.*
- Some common things that children are allergic to include
  ~ Foods, especially peanuts, tree nuts, soy, milk, wheat, eggs, fish, and shellfish
  ~ Pollen
  ~ Mold or mildew
  ~ Dust mites
  ~ Animal dander, especially from cats and dogs
  ~ Inhaled scents (Perfume, incense, and smoke are irritants that cause symptoms, but not allergens.)
  ~ Medications
  ~ Topicals (things that are placed on the skin such as creams or lotions)
  ~ Insect stings or droppings
  ~ Latex

How common is it?

Allergies are very common. In a national study of children with special health care needs, 53% had allergies of some type.

What adaptations may be needed?

Dietary considerations

- See Anaphylaxis on page 61 for more information about dietary adaptations for allergic conditions.
- Some children will have mild allergies to food and do not require strict controls.

Physical environment

- Include teaching about allergies in the educational curriculum. Make a game of allergy symptoms and body parts (eg, watery eyes, stuffy nose, skin rash). Learning about allergies can also be an opportunity to see the ways that our bodies interact with the world (eg, touching, smelling, tasting).
- Post lists of the children's allergies in a place that staff can see but the public and other children cannot.
- Always consider using hypoallergenic products such as soaps and cleaning products.
- Change air filters frequently to cut down on airborne allergens.
- Ask parents/guardians to be specific about their child's allergy. People tend to use the term loosely. Find out which allergies are serious and which cause minor problems.
- Allergies can change over time. Ask parents/guardians to keep their child's Care Plan updated with respect to allergies.

What are some related Quick Reference Sheets?

- Allergic Skin Conditions (page 53)
- Anaphylaxis (page 61)
- Asthma (page 65)

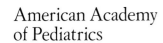

American Academy of Pediatrics

DEDICATED TO THE HEALTH OF ALL CHILDREN™

Altered Immunity: An Overview

What is altered immunity?

- The immune system helps to protect the body from infections and cancers.
- The immune system is very complex and requires many parts to work well together. When one piece of the puzzle is missing, some parts of the immune system may work and others might not function adequately.
- Causes of an abnormal immune system include
  ~ HIV
  ~ Genetic condition—B- or T-cell deficiencies (present at birth)
  ~ Steroids or other medications, such as cancer treatment, that suppress the immune system
  ~ Chronic illness—nephrotic syndrome, diabetes, metabolic diseases
  ~ Spleen problem—missing or not working properly (eg, spleen removed after trauma or sickle cell disease)
  ~ Cancer treatment—a low white blood cell count
  ~ Transplantation—organ or bone marrow

How common is it?

No one knows for sure how many children have suppressed immune systems. It is becoming more common as more children receive transplants and survive serious problems with their immune systems like HIV. Some children have temporary alterations in their immune system from medications and the immune system returns to normal when the medication is stopped.

What are some characteristics of children with altered immunity?

- There are a few common characteristics for children with immune problems. Some of the infections that tend to be the biggest problems are infections such as pneumonia, chickenpox, measles, and herpes cold sores.
  ~ Measles and chickenpox vaccines have drastically reduced the number of cases of those diseases.
  ~ However, there are still cases of chickenpox that occur (breakthrough cases) and they can be missed because they are so mild. Most of the time, this is not a problem for children with healthy immune systems, but it can be a problem for children with an altered or a weakened immune system.

~ It is important that all children who come into contact with an immune-suppressed child be vaccinated against measles and chickenpox.
~ Children with altered immunity should avoid direct exposure to the lesions of a child or caregiver with an active cold sore.
- Fever is a serious sign in children with immune problems and should be evaluated immediately. Most parents/guardians recognize this and will seek treatment for their child promptly.
- Because there are so many reasons a child could have an immune system problem, it is possible that the child could enter child care or school with the diagnosis or develop it while enrolled. The immune problem can occur for a short time, such as with children on steroids for a few weeks, or it can occur for a long time, such as with children with transplants.

What adaptations may be needed?

Medications

Some children will have enough of a problem responding to even weakened viruses that they cannot safely receive live-virus vaccines. Such children will have medical records that document their medical exemption from live-virus vaccines that excuse them from regulatory requirements for these specific vaccines (ie, varicella, measles). They will only receive vaccines that do not contain live material.

Physical environment

Adaptations for immune suppression depend on the specific disease. It is important to have a complete and up-to-date Care Plan that is reviewed with the child's parents/guardians.

What should be considered an emergency?

- Fever is usually an emergency for a child with a suppressed immune system.
- It is critical that emergency medical services/911 first responders know that the child has an immune problem.

What types of training or polices are advised?

Staff should recognize the need for prompt action for fever.

➤*continued*

Altered Immunity: An Overview, continued

What are some related Quick Reference Sheets?

- Cancer (page 75)
- Diabetes (page 85)
- Human Immunodeficiency Virus (HIV) (page 109)
- Kidney/Urinary Problems (page 115)
- Special Diets and Inborn Errors of Metabolism (page 129)
- Spleen Problems (page 133)

American Academy
of Pediatrics

DEDICATED TO THE HEALTH OF ALL CHILDREN™

Anaphylaxis

What is anaphylaxis?

- Anaphylaxis is a life-threatening allergic reaction that affects the whole body. It happens when the body has an intense response to an allergen. Symptoms can include
  ~ Drop in blood pressure
  ~ Flushing, sweating, or paleness of the skin
  ~ Swelling of the skin, lips, mouth, or throat
  ~ Raised red rash (hives) and itching
  ~ Nausea or stomach cramps
  ~ Difficulty breathing, including wheezing
  ~ Fainting, light-headedness, or convulsions
  ~ Cardiorespiratory arrest
- These symptoms usually occur within minutes of contact with the allergen or allergy-causing substance; however, sometimes symptoms can be delayed a few hours.
- Anaphylaxis can be caused by many things, but insect stings, food (especially nuts), medications, and latex are some of the more common allergens.

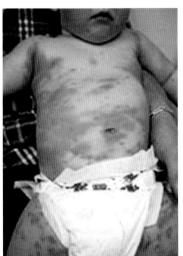

Swelling caused by an allergic reaction

PETE SMITH, MD

How common is it?

- Anaphylaxis occurs in 30 out of 100,000 persons.
- Food allergy occurs in between 2% and 8% of children.

What are some characteristics of children with anaphylaxis?

- Anaphylaxis usually occurs with no warning, although it can happen more frequently in children with other known allergies.

- A child may come to your child care program or school with a diagnosis of being at risk for anaphylaxis, or the child may develop the condition while enrolled.

Who is the treatment team?

- The primary care provider in the medical home is the major point of contact.
- Allergists may also be important team members.
- Consider contacting local emergency medical services (EMS)/911 providers for questions about planning for emergencies.

What adaptations may be needed?

Medications

- Anaphylaxis is treated with injected epinephrine, which is commonly packaged in an automatically injected device like EpiPen or EpiPen Jr. The pen is pressed against the skin (usually the thigh) and activated.
- Always call EMS/911 when injected epinephrine is used.
- Always call parents/guardians and tell them what hospital the child has been transported to.
- Injected epinephrine is effective for 15 to 20 minutes. It may need to be used a second time if EMS/911 are not able to respond quickly.
  ~ Side effects of epinephrine include pallor, vomiting, fast heart rate, and jitteriness.

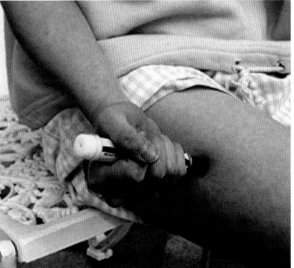

How to administer an EpiPen

ALLERGY CAPITAL

➤continued

- There may be instructions to use other medications as well for allergies such as diphenhydramine (Benadryl is one brand name).
  - ~ Side effects of diphenhydramine include sleepiness, but some children may experience excitement.
- All medications should be properly stored. Procedures should be in place to check expiration dates and obtain fresh medication as needed.
- Staff training on EpiPen and Benadryl use is very important.

Dietary considerations

- Avoiding foods that cause anaphylaxis for the involved child is crucial. Some foods that are common allergens include peanuts, tree nuts, soy, eggs, and milk. It is not easy to avoid peanuts because peanut oil is in many products. Cross contamination can occur when foods are processed and packaged. Strategies include starting a table that has whatever food restriction is necessary or making the classroom and any other areas the child uses free of the allergen. In some cases, strict hand-washing precautions after eating or avoiding the offending food must involve all the children who share the spaces that the allergic child uses to protect the allergic child from exposure to the allergen while at the child care or school. Even touching a surface touched by a child who has had contact with the allergen can be sufficient to cause a reaction for very sensitive children. Using specially marked place mats to remind caregivers which child has a food allergy can be helpful, but it does not stop children from sharing food.
- In some cases, it is best for parents/guardians to supply food for the child with the allergy. In other cases, the child care/school staff may be able to provide food as long as they have been fully educated about avoiding specific food allergens.
- A policy about accepting foods from parents/guardians should be maintained (see *Caring for Our Children: National Health and Safety Performance Standards: Guidelines for Out-of-Home Child Care Programs,* 2nd Edition, Standard 4.040). Parents/guardians of all the children in the child's class should be advised to avoid any known allergens in any treats that they supply to the class.
- Store-bought or commercial products are acceptable as long as the package list of ingredients is provided. Parents of children with food allergies are usually very willing to take time to read these ingredients to ensure the safety of their children.
- The American Academy of Allergy, Asthma & Immunology position paper, "Anaphylaxis in Schools and Other Child-Care Settings" (www.aaaai.org/members/ academy_statements/position_statements/ps34.asp), states, "…handwashing after food handling should be encouraged in day care and preschool settings, as well as in lower schools." Soap and warm water should be sufficient for washing (see *Caring for Our Children,* 2nd Edition, standards 3.020–3.021).
- A list of children with any known allergies should be posted where it can be easily seen by staff but not by the public and other children.

Physical environment

The key adaptation to avoiding anaphylaxis is to try to avoid the allergen. This may mean
- Avoiding products with latex or those with strong perfumes.
- Being extra cautious during outside play if stinging insects are around, and avoiding eating outside. Encourage closed-toe shoes in children with known allergies.
- Avoiding food allergens. In some cases, just physical contact with the food can cause a reaction even if the child doesn't eat it.

Transportation considerations

- Injectable epinephrine should be available as the child is transported to and from child care or school. For field trips, the injectable epinephrine and someone who can administer it should be available. A mobile phone and a copy of the child's Care Plan should be carried at all times.
- In emergency evacuation situations, injectable epinephrine should be carried.

What should be considered an emergency?

- Early symptoms of anaphylaxis can include hoarse voice, sore throat, or feeling of throat closing or tingling. Other common symptoms include skin or mouth swelling, a feeling of panic, and stomach cramps or vomiting. Difficulty breathing or wheezing are serious symptoms as well. The child may be pale or dizzy.
- Children who are stung by an insect should be monitored closely for symptoms of anaphylaxis.
- If symptoms of anaphylaxis are present, call EMS/911 immediately. Inject epinephrine if available and keep the child relaxed and in the position of greatest comfort.
- If symptoms do not improve after 10 minutes or if symptoms return, a second dose of epinephrine can be given if EMS/911 first responders have not yet arrived.
- Be prepared to start CPR if the child stops breathing.

➤continued

Anaphylaxis, continued

- If the child has a symptom about which you are unsure, call the parent/guardian immediately and prepare to give injectable epinephrine if necessary.
- Parents/guardians should be notified of any possible exposure to an allergen even if a reaction did not occur.

What types of training or policies are advised?

- Care Plan outlining specific instructions.
- Avoiding food allergens.
- Recognizing anaphylaxis.
- Responding to anaphylaxis.
- The Food Allergy & Anaphylaxis Network Web site (www.foodallergy.org) has great training information.
- Some pharmaceutical companies also have good training materials.
- Consider having a health consultant give a training presentation.
- A policy on food allergies should be written.

What are some resources?

- Food Allergy & Anaphylaxis Network, 11781 Lee Jackson Hwy, Suite 160, Fairfax, VA 22033-3309; 800/929-4040; www.foodallergy.org
- American Academy of Allergy, Asthma & Immunology, www.aaaai.org
- American Academy of Pediatrics, American Public Health Association, National Resource Center for Health and Safety in Child Care. Standard 4.009: feeding plans. In: American Academy of Pediatrics, American Public Health Association, National Resource Center for Health and Safety in Child Care. *Caring for Our Children: National Health and Safety Performance Standards: Guidelines for Out-of-Home Child Care Programs.* 2nd ed. Elk Grove Village, IL: American Academy of Pediatrics; 2002:153–154
- American Academy of Pediatrics, American Public Health Association, National Resource Center for Health and Safety in Child Care. Standard 4.010: care for children with food allergies. In: American Academy of Pediatrics, American Public Health Association, National Resource Center for Health and Safety in Child Care. *Caring for Our Children: National Health and Safety Performance Standards: Guidelines for Out-of-Home Child Care Programs.* 2nd ed. Elk Grove Village, IL: American Academy of Pediatrics; 2002:154–155

American Academy of Pediatrics

DEDICATED TO THE HEALTH OF ALL CHILDREN™

American Academy of Pediatrics
Web site — www.aap.org

Asthma

What is asthma?

- Asthma is a chronic long-term condition in which air passages to the lungs become inflamed, swollen, and narrowed. The swelling can narrow passages enough to reduce or block airflow to and from the lungs. As air moves through the narrowed airway, it can make a wheezing sound.
- Children with asthma may have repeated episodes of wheezing, breathlessness, and chest tightness with nighttime or early morning coughing.

How common is it?

Asthma is one of the most common chronic diseases in children, affecting between 5% and 10%.

What are some characteristics of children with asthma?

- Asthma can vary from mild to severe and it can be occasional or continuous.
- Asthma can worsen with infections, weather changes, or exposure to an asthma trigger. Asthma triggers are those things that make asthma worse. Common triggers include viral infections, smoke, dust, mold, dust mites, cockroaches, and animal dander.
- Children with asthma may cough, wheeze, or have no symptoms at all depending on how much air is moving at that time. Cough can be one of the first symptoms that the child experiences when asthma is acting up. Wheezing that can be heard also means there is a problem.
- If the child's airway is badly blocked, nothing might be heard, but the child will look like she is having trouble breathing.
- Asthma can and should be controlled. A child whose asthma is under control will look like any other child, be able to play normally, and only rarely have asthma symptoms. This is one of the goals of asthma care—to have the child live a normal life. Luckily, with good asthma care, this is possible for most children with asthma.
- A key component of good asthma control is management education for parents and self-management education for older school-aged children. Caregivers/teachers should support older children in self-managing their asthma, which includes recognizing symptoms and permitting those children with adequate knowledge, skills, and behaviors to carry and administer quick-relief medication (see "When Should Students With Asthma or Allergies Carry and Self-Administer Emergency Medications at School?" in Chapter 11 on page 173).

- Children who require frequent quick-relief medication for symptoms may need better controller medications. Use of quick-relief medication and any symptoms that keep children from fully participating in activities should be documented. This information is important to give to parents/guardians so they can share it with the child's prescribing health care professional.

What are some elements of a Care Plan for asthma?

- The Asthma Action Plan is a specialized Care Plan for children with asthma.
- Asthma Action Plans should include a list of the child's asthma triggers and which things to avoid. It should be updated after hospitalizations, emergency visits, child absences for illness, and changes in medications. Samples of Asthma Action Plans can be found in Chapter 11.
- Asthma Action Plans are usually designed with 3 zones based on a traffic light—red, yellow, and green.
  - **Green zone** is the plan when the child is doing well and includes any controller medications that the child needs to take to stay healthy (see "Medications").
  - **Yellow zone** outlines the plan if the child begins to develop symptoms such as cough and the plan for quick-relief medications (see "Medications").
  - **Red zone** is the trouble area when the child needs prompt and vigorous treatment.
- Older children may use a peak flow meter to monitor their airway health. Peak flow numbers can be used to determine when children should take their quick-relief medication and to monitor how they are doing at different times of the day.

What adaptations may be needed?

Medications

- Asthma medications are often categorized as *controller* or *quick relief.* These 2 types are used together for better asthma control.
- Controller medications
  - Fight the inflammation and keep the airways open.
  - The most common controller medications are inhaled steroids, which are typically given by parents/guardians at home.
  - There are few side effects of these medications, but the mouth should be rinsed after taking inhaled steroids to avoid thrush, a yeast infection of the mouth lining.
  - Sometimes the child will take oral steroids, like prednisone, by mouth for a short period.

➤continued

Asthma, continued

~ Side effects of oral steroids include mood swings, increased appetite, nausea, weight gain, and behavior changes. If taken over a longer period, the immune system can be suppressed.
- Quick-relief medications
  ~ Relieve the muscle spasm to allow better airflow on a temporary basis.
  ~ Sometimes are referred to as *rescue* medications, but this terminology is not preferred because it can imply waiting until symptoms are bad.
  ~ The most common quick-relief medications are beta agonists such as albuterol. Side effects include jitteriness, fast heart rate, and hyperactivity. Some children will be sleepy after a treatment.
  ~ Albuterol can be administered in different ways.
    ❖ Nebulizers—machines that drive air through liquid medication and make it into a mist that can be inhaled. Typically it takes 5 to 10 minutes to complete a treatment using a nebulizer.
      - Younger children may use a mask over their mouth and nose to get medication; older children may breathe through a mouthpiece.
      - The delivery device and its tubing should be cleaned regularly and dried completely.
      - Some children dislike nebulizer treatments and may need a distraction such as reading a book or watching a video.
    ❖ Metered-dose inhalers and spacers—most people lack the coordination to properly use a metered-dose inhaler and will get a better dose of medication if they use a spacer device. Typically, the child must have the device placed properly and then take several breaths to complete the treatment.
  ~ Quick-relief medications should be available for children with asthma to use if they need it while they are at school or child care.
  ~ The ways to recognize that the child needs treatment with a quick-relief medication should be clearly stated in lay language in the Care Plan (see Sample Asthma Action Plan in Chapter 11 on page 167).
- As always, expiration dates of medications should be checked regularly and medications should be stored in a safe location. The number of puffs used should be documented and a cumulative count kept, ensuring that medication is still in the inhaler.
- Children with asthma are especially vulnerable to respiratory infections. All children should get a flu shot every year, but especially those with asthma.

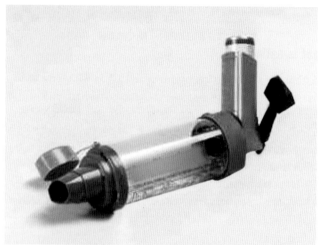
Metered-dose inhaler

ASTHMA AND ALLERGY FOUNDATION OF AMERICA

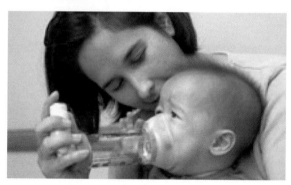
Inhaler with spacer for asthma medications

ANDREW SILK

Dietary considerations

Diet may need to be modified for children with asthma who have food allergies.

Physical environment

- Indoor environment—be tobacco free; control mold and mildew by fixing any water leak quickly; avoid furry or feathered pets; clean frequently; use integrated pest management to limit pesticide use and pests; use dust covers for bedding; ensure good ventilation; change air filters frequently; and avoid strong perfumes or scented cleaning products.
- Outdoor play—be aware of ozone and pollen levels. Extremes of air temperature can sometimes be a problem but should be balanced with the child's need to run and play outdoors. These are good issues to problem solve with parents/guardians and health care professionals. Children with exercise-induced asthma may need to use their albuterol inhaler before physical activity.

➤*continued*

Asthma, continued

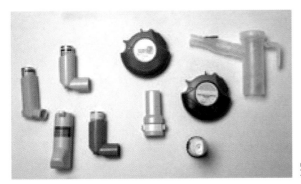

Devices for asthma medication

AAP

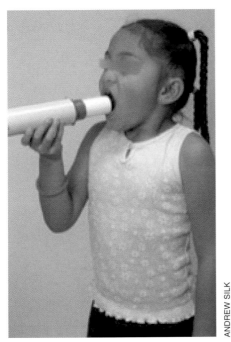

ANDREW SILK

A peak flow meter measures how fast a person can blow air out of the lungs.

Transportation considerations

- Consider how to handle respiratory distress that develops during transportation to and from school or child care settings if transportation is not done by parents.
- If the child's asthma is temperature sensitive, be aware of vehicle temperatures and take time to use heat or air conditioning to stabilize the temperature as necessary before the child enters the vehicle.

What should be considered an emergency?

- Notify parents/guardians if
  - ~ Symptoms do not improve with one dose of prescribed quick-relief medication.
  - ~ Two or more doses of quick-relief medication have been needed during the day.
- Always notify parents about any asthma symptoms, even when they do not reach the level that constitutes an emergency, so that parents can work with the child's health care professional to monitor the control of the child's asthma and keep the symptoms under good control. A daily symptom checklist can be a good communication tool to use with parents.
- Call emergency medical services/911 for
  - ~ Severe breathing problems such as struggling to breathe, or pulling in at the neck or under the rib cage with every breath.
  - ~ Child is having difficulty talking or walking.
  - ~ Lips or fingernails are turning blue.
  - ~ Symptoms are not improving after a second dose of quick-relief medication.
- Keep emergency contact information updated at all times.

What types of training or policies are advised?

- Preventing exposure of the child to asthma triggers.
- Recognizing the symptoms of an acute asthma episode.
- Treating acute episodes including the purpose of treatment, expected response, and possible side effects. Caregivers should be able to assist and supervise the child during the treatment.
- Using health consultants for training.
- Look for asthma coalitions in your area.
- Work as a team.
- Track absences and early dismissals.
- There should be a clear policy about exclusion and readmission for active wheezing.

➤continued

Asthma, continued

What are some resources?

- American Academy of Pediatrics, American Public Health Association, National Resource Center for Health and Safety in Child Care. Standard 3.062: management of children with asthma. In: American Academy of Pediatrics, American Public Health Association, National Resource Center for Health and Safety in Child Care. *Caring for Our Children: National Health and Safety Performance Standards: Guidelines for Out-of-Home Child Care Programs.* 2nd ed. Elk Grove Village, IL: American Academy of Pediatrics; 2002:120–122
- National Asthma Education and Prevention Program and National Heart, Lung, and Blood Institute, www.nhlbi.nih.gov/health/prof/lung (look under "Asthma Materials for Schools")
  - ~ How Asthma-Friendly Is Your Child-Care Setting? (www.nhlbi.nih.gov/health/public/lung/asthma/chc_chk.pdf)
  - ~ How Asthma-Friendly Is Your School? (www.nhlbi.nih.gov/health/public/lung/asthma/friendly.pdf)
  - ~ *Managing Asthma: A Guide for Schools* (2003 Edition) (www.nhlbi.nih.gov/health/prof/lung/asthma/asth_sch.pdf)

- US Environmental Protection Agency, *Indoor Air Quality (IAQ) Tools for Schools,* www.epa.gov/iaq/schools
- Centers for Disease Control and Prevention, www.cdc.gov/HealthyYouth/asthma/strategies.htm
- Asthma and Allergy Foundation of America, www.aafa.org
- American Lung Association, www.lungusa.org/site/pp.asp?c=dvLUK9O0E&b=22542
- National Institute of Allergy and Infectious Diseases, www3.niaid.nih.gov

American Academy of Pediatrics

DEDICATED TO THE HEALTH OF ALL CHILDREN™

Attention-Deficit/Hyperactivity Disorder (ADHD)

What is attention-deficit/hyperactivity disorder (ADHD)?

- Attention-deficit/hyperactivity disorder (ADHD) is a behavior disorder characterized by attention problems and/or hyperactivity and impulsivity.
- Attention-deficit/hyperactivity disorder is usually diagnosed in childhood. The symptoms of ADHD, when present, are almost always apparent in some form by the age of 7 years.
- The type of ADHD that just involves inattention may not be evident until a child is expected to meet some of the higher expectations of third or fourth grade.

How common is it?

- Estimates suggest that between 3% and 9% of all children have ADHD.
- It is more common in boys than in girls, with the ratio estimated at approximately 4:1.

What are some characteristics of children with ADHD?

- Many children, especially preschoolers, can appear very energetic, active, and impulsive.
- In children with ADHD, the symptoms of inattention, impulsivity, and hyperactivity are more extreme. These symptoms interfere with learning, school or preschool adjustment, and the child's relationship with family and friends. These symptoms may persist through adolescence and into adulthood. The most common symptoms of ADHD include
  - ~ Inattention
    - ❖ Short attention span for age
    - ❖ Difficulty listening to others
    - ❖ Difficulty attending to details
    - ❖ Easily distracted
    - ❖ Poor organizational or study skills for age
    - ❖ Forgetful
  - ~ Impulsivity
    - ❖ Often interrupts others.
    - ❖ Has difficulty waiting for his turn in school or social games.
    - ❖ Acts before thinking; often takes risks.
    - ❖ Tends to blurt out answers instead of waiting to be called on.
  - ~ Hyperactivity
    - ❖ Always in motion, as if "driven by a motor."
    - ❖ Has difficulty remaining in her seat even when it is expected.
    - ❖ Fidgets with hands or squirms when in her seat.
    - ❖ Talks excessively.
    - ❖ Has difficulty engaging in quiet activities.
    - ❖ Inability to stay on task; shifts from one task to another without bringing any to completion.
- Attention-deficit/hyperactivity disorder is the most commonly diagnosed behavior disorder of childhood.
  - ~ The diagnosis can be made by the primary care provider in the medical home, developmental-behavioral pediatrician, child psychiatrist, neurologist, psychologist, or qualified mental health professional.
  - ~ A detailed history of the child's behavior from parents and teachers, a physical examination, and observations of the child's behavior contribute to making the diagnosis of ADHD.
  - ~ Psychological or educational testing may help define co-occurring behavioral or learning disabilities.

Who is the treatment team?

- The treatment team for children with ADHD includes their primary care provider in the medical home, parents, teachers, mental health professionals, educational specialists, and other professionals who are involved with an individual child.
- Treatment should include education for children and their families, as well as behavior and medication management if indicated.
- Primary care providers should also establish a long-term plan for systemic follow-up support (a medical home), as with any chronic condition.

What are some elements of a Care Plan for ADHD?

Behavior management skills that can be included in a Care Plan include
- Praise for appropriate behaviors that are being worked on
- Using active ignoring when undesired behaviors occur that are not dangerous or intolerable
- Using praise and ignoring in combination with each other
- Point or token systems for behavior rewards and consequences

➤continued

Attention-Deficit/Hyperactivity Disorder (ADHD), continued

- Preferential seating in a classroom to decrease distraction
- Daily report cards or communication logs to travel between home and school

What adaptations may be needed?

Medications

- Medication for ADHD is used for the purpose of balancing chemicals in the brain to help the child maintain attention and control impulses.
- Stimulant medications are the most frequently used medications for ADHD. There are short-acting (4-hour), intermediate-acting (6- to 8-hour), and long-acting (12-hour) stimulant medications.
- Some children require a medication dose during school or child care.
- These medications may have side effects including decreased appetite, trouble sleeping or napping, headache, or stomachache.

Physical environment

- Children with ADHD may be eligible for accommodations in school or child care through Section 504 of the Rehabilitation Act of 1973. This may allow a child preferential seating in the classroom, the ability to take a test in a quiet room, or other structures and supports that will allow him to succeed in school or child care.
- If ADHD symptoms significantly interfere with learning, an Individualized Education Program can be requested as part of the Individuals With Disabilities Education Act.
- Develop strategies for accommodating children with ADHD. Suggestions include
  - ~ Provide children with a consistent routine to the day and structure to the environment. Let them know when the routine is changing or something unusual is going to happen, such as a class trip or a special visitor.
  - ~ Give the child clear boundaries and expectations. These instructions and guidelines are best given right before the activity or situation.

- ~ Devise an appropriate reward system for good behavior or completing a certain number of positive behaviors, such as a merit-point or gold-star program with a specific reward, like a favorite activity. The strongest rewards are often "Good job!" right at the time that the positive behavior occurs.
- ~ Avoid using food and especially candy for rewards.
- ~ Use a timer for activities to build and reinforce structure.
- ~ As much as possible, give clear instructions and explanations for tasks throughout the day. If a task is complex or lengthy, break it down into steps.
- ~ Communicate regularly with the child's parents/guardians so that behaviors can be addressed before they become disruptive.
- ~ Children with ADHD need role models for behavior more than other children, and the adults in their lives are very important in this regard.

What should be considered an emergency?

- Attention-deficit/hyperactivity disorder does not have any specific emergencies associated with it.
- Emergencies may occur if an overdose of medication is given. Call parents if a known overdose of medication is given at school or child care, or for sudden erratic changes in a child's behavior.
- Emergency medical services/911 should be called if a child on medication becomes overly drowsy or lethargic.

What are some resources?

- *Caring for Children With ADHD: A Resource Toolkit for Clinicians,* American Academy of Pediatrics, www.aap.org/bookstore, 888/227-1770
- Children and Adults with Attention Deficit/Hyperactivity Disorder, 8181 Professional Place, Suite 150, Landover, MD 20785, 800/233-4050, 301/306-7090 (fax), www.chadd.org

American Academy of Pediatrics

DEDICATED TO THE HEALTH OF ALL CHILDREN™

Autism Spectrum Disorders

What are autism spectrum disorders?

Autism spectrum disorders (ASDs) are a group of developmental disabilities caused by a problem with the brain. Children with ASDs have trouble in 3 core areas of their development.
- Language difficulties, especially no apparent desire to communicate
- Social interactions
- Restricted interests or behaviors that are repeated over and over again (known as *stereotyped* behaviors)

How common are they?

- Recent statistics estimate that as many as 1 in 150 children may be diagnosed with an ASD.
- Approximately 24,000 children are diagnosed with an ASD each year, with an estimate of 500,000 children aged 0 to 21 years with an ASD.
- Autism spectrum disorders occur more frequently in boys than girls.

What are some characteristics of children with autism spectrum disorders?

- Children with an ASD often look similar to other children, but they may communicate, interact, behave, and learn in ways that are different.
- These children may have problems with social, emotional, and communication skills.
- Children with an ASD might
  ~ Avoid eye contact.
  ~ Fail to respond to their names when called.
  ~ Fail to look in the direction of interesting objects pointed out to them and not point themselves (this is called a *joint-attention deficit*).
  ~ Move away from others or may not interact with them.
  ~ Echo words or phrases in place of normal language (this is called *echolalia*).
  ~ Repeat actions such as rocking, hand flapping, or handling an object in the same way over and over again.
  ~ Regress in their development or lose skills they once had, such as language.
  ~ Have difficulty communicating and expressing their own needs.
  ~ Become upset when things change or when it is time to transition to a new activity.
  ~ Have unusual reactions to sensory stimuli (eg, smells, tastes, sounds, touches). This can range from trying to block out the stimulus to not responding to pain or something that others find scary or dangerous.

- Prior to diagnosis, parents/guardians and caregivers/teaches may observe signs of an ASD. These children may
  ~ Play with toys in an inappropriate manner (eg, lining cars up instead of driving them around).
  ~ Not have an appropriate gaze.
  ~ Lack warm, joyful expressions with gaze.
  ~ Lack the alternating to-and-fro pattern of vocalizations between infant and parent that usually occurs at approximately 6 months of age (ie, infants with ASDs usually continue vocalizing without regard for the parent/guardian's speech).
  ~ Not recognize their parent/guardian's or caregiver/teacher's voice.
  ~ Have disregard for vocalizations (eg, lack of response to name), yet keen awareness for environmental sounds.
  ~ Have delayed onset of babbling past 9 months of age.
  ~ Have decreased or absent use of pre-speech gestures (eg, waving, pointing, showing).
  ~ Lack expressions such as "Oh oh" or "Huh."
  ~ Not demonstrate interest or response of any kind to neutral statements (eg, "Oh no, it's raining again!")

Who is the treatment team?

The treatment team for children with ASDs can include a primary care provider in the medical home, a developmental pediatrician, a pediatric neurologist, a child psychiatrist, a child psychologist, and speech and occupational therapists.

What are some elements of a Care Plan for autism spectrum disorders?

- The main research-based treatment for ASDs is intensive structured teaching of skills, often called *behavioral intervention.* There are many different interventions, including those taught to the child's parents, that are useful.
- *Speech therapy* is often a part of the Care Plan of a child with an ASD because speech is often delayed. Children with an ASD need to learn how to communicate using language and nonverbal skills. Speech therapists address deficits in joint attention as a first step in teaching oral language. They may also use picture exchange boards, signing, or typing as a bridge to oral communication with these children.
- *Occupational therapy* may help children learn self-help and manipulative skills as well as how to accept and respond more typically to sounds, smells, and touch.

➤*continued*

Autism Spectrum Disorders, continued

- Children who are younger than 3 years may receive their therapies through *early intervention* services. Early intervention is a system of services to support infants and toddlers with disabilities and their families.
- Children 3 years or older may receive *special education and related services* through the public schools. The behavioral intervention is designed to help children with ASDs succeed in school.

What adaptations may be needed?

Medications

- Medications may be used to help a child with an ASD control anxiety, obsessions, hyperactivity, or aggression.
- Talk to the child's parents about any medications that the child might be taking and what side effects might occur with those medications. See Chapter 6 for more information about medication administration.

Dietary considerations

- There are many nonproven dietary treatments for ASDs that may not be directed by the child's treatment team.
- Families of children with ASDs may use gluten- and casein-free diets, medication to treat yeast, and vitamins, although there is no medical evidence to support their use and some may be dangerous.
- Programs should develop and discuss with families their policies about implementing special instructions that are not part of a medically recommended Care Plan. In general, any such instructions that a program is inclined to include for a child should be reviewed with the child's health care professional to be sure they do not pose risks of injury or illness for the child or staff.

Physical environment

Classroom placement and teacher selection—choosing a supportive classroom environment is very important. The caregiver/teacher, other children in the group, and room layout should be selected so that everyone can have their own needs met.

- Structure helps the child with an ASD understand his surroundings and what is expected of him. Structure is a form of behavioral management that helps children with ASDs be calmer, less agitated, and more successful with learning. Some helpful structure tools can be
  - ~ Classroom organization and arrangement
  - ~ Individual daily schedules

- ~ Individual work systems
- ~ Visual charts
- In addition, it is important to know that children with an ASD
  - ~ Can and do form emotional attachments, although there is an impairment in these relationships.
  - ~ Have characteristics and behaviors that often improve as a result of intervention, but do not outgrow and are not cured of an ASD.
  - ~ Have uneven learning and cognitive skills.
  - ~ May have some degree of intellectual disability (about 50% have an intellectual disability).
  - ~ Often have difficulty with understanding instructions and can develop confusion and anxiety, resulting in a behavioral outburst that is misinterpreted as noncompliance.
  - ~ Come from families of all races and socioeconomic backgrounds.
  - ~ Often will require varying levels of support to maintain a home and job as they become adults.

What should be considered an emergency?

There are no special medical emergencies to which children with ASDs are prone, but they may need extra time and supervision in the event of a programmatic emergency such as a fire. This should be taken into consideration in emergency planning.

What are some resources?

- American Academy of Pediatrics, www.aap.org/healthtopics/autism.cfm
- *Caring for Children With Autism Spectrum Disorders: A Resource Toolkit for Clinicians,* American Academy of Pediatrics, www.aap.org/bookstore, 888/227-1770
- Autism Society of America, 7910 Woodmont Ave, Suite 300, Bethesda, MD 20814-3067, 800/3AUTISM (328-8476), www.autism-society.org
- National Dissemination Center for Children with Disabilities, 800/695-0285 (voice/TTY), www.nichcy.org
- Autism Spectrum Disorders Fact Sheet, Centers for Disease Control and Prevention, 800/CDC-INFO (232-4636), www.cdc.gov/actearly
- Autism Speaks, www.autismspeaks.org
- First Signs, Inc, www.firstsigns.org

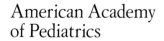

American Academy of Pediatrics

DEDICATED TO THE HEALTH OF ALL CHILDREN™

Bleeding Disorders: An Overview

What are bleeding disorders?

- *Bleeding disorders* is a general term to describe medical conditions in which the blood does not clot well.
- The process of blood clotting is very complex and things can go wrong at many stages. There are 2 parts of the blood that are required for effective clotting—tiny cells in the blood called *platelets* and proteins called *clotting factors*. When blood does not clot, the child may bruise easily, have nosebleeds, or bleed for a long time after being injured or after surgery.
- Platelet problems
  - ~ Having a low platelet count can interfere with normal clotting. Low platelet counts can be caused by different diseases or as a side effect of certain medications.
  - ~ The most common disease causing low platelets is idiopathic thrombocytopenic purpura (ITP). See "Idiopathic Thrombocytopenic Purpura" on page 113 for more details.
  - ~ There are also rare disorders of platelet function that can have similar bleeding tendencies.
- Clotting factor disorders
  - ~ The 2 most common of these disorders are von Willebrand disease and hemophilia.
  - ~ Von Willebrand disease can affect males and females equally, but hemophilia usually only affects males.

How common are they?

- Statistics about von Willebrand disease vary depending on whether very mild cases are included. Some think the condition may be as common as 1% to 2% of the population, but others feel that it affects only 1 in 1,000 people (0.1%).
- Hemophilia occurs in 1 in 5,000 male births and affects approximately 18,000 people, mostly male, in the United States.

What are some characteristics of children with bleeding disorders?

- Bleeding disorders may cause lumps under the skin (hematomas) or flat collections of pinpoint bleeding in the skin called *petechiae.*
- Spontaneous bleeding or bleeding after trauma can occur in the joints or the intestinal and urinary tracks.
- Nosebleeds and bleeding from the gums or teeth may also be common.
- Hemophilia

  - ~ Deeper and surgical bleeding is more common in hemophilia. Bleeding into the joints can cause problems over time for children with hemophilia; efforts are made to avoid this complication.
  - ~ Children with hemophilia are often treated with infusion of the missing clotting factors. In the past, these clotting factors were derived from blood and placed children with hemophilia at risk for blood-borne infections such as hepatitis B and C and HIV, but changes in the way clotting factors are produced have reduced this problem. Since the mid to late 1980s, treatment of these blood-clotting factors as well as the use of genetically engineered clotting factors have essentially eliminated the risk of blood-borne infections.
- Von Willebrand disease
  - ~ Usually presents with more superficial bleeding such as nose, mouth, and menstrual.
  - ~ Can vary in severity, but most forms cause less serious bleeding than hemophilia.

Who is the treatment team?

- Children with hemophilia and von Willebrand disease require specialty care. The physicians who care for them are called hematologists and they manage them along with other specialty nurses, physical therapists, and social workers as well as the primary care provider in the medical home.
- Children with von Willebrand disease bleed less than children with hemophilia and therefore need less urgent and frequent specialty care, but hematologists are usually involved in the care of their bleeding problems prior to surgery or procedures, or after trauma.

What adaptations may be needed?

Bleeding disorders vary in types and severity, so it is best to get details about the specific child's needs from parents/guardians and the child's specialty doctors.

Medications

- A medication called desmopressin acetate (DDAVP) can help prevent or eliminate bleeding in some types of bleeding disorders. It can be given by injection or sprayed into the nose.
- Some children with a more severe form of hemophilia will have a long-term intravenous catheter placed so they can get treated with clotting factors more easily.

➤*continued*

Bleeding Disorders: An Overview, continued

- All children with clotting disorders should avoid nonsteroidal anti-inflammatory drugs such as ibuprofen (eg, Advil, Motrin), naproxen (eg, Aleve), and aspirin.
- Acetaminophen (eg, Tylenol) is usually fine to use, but patients with bleeding disorders should discuss any medications to be taken, even over-the-counter medicines, with their hematologist.

Dietary considerations

There is no special diet for bleeding disorders, but it is important that the child not become overweight because that can put more stress on the joints.

Physical environment

- Avoiding trauma, especially to the head, can be a big challenge, particularly in the preschool years. Be extra cautious that straps in high chairs are fastened and that children are watched carefully on elevated surfaces such as changing tables and when climbing. Pad any sharp corners. Some children with severe hemophilia may wear helmets to protect their heads, but this is not common and is usually done to reduce the risk of further bleeding in a child who has already suffered a head bleed. Gym activities may need to be adapted for school-aged children.
- First aid—cool compresses can be used for bleeding. Popsicles are sometimes helpful for mouth injuries, but don't allow the child to keep the popsicle in one place for too long to avoid cold injury.
- If a nosebleed occurs, pinch the end of the nose below the nasal bone for 10 minutes and have the child stay in a neutral position. Some children with mild von Willebrand disease do not need any special adaptations, just awareness of their condition in case they are injured or require emergency treatment.
- Exercises such as bicycle riding, walking, and swimming are good ways to keep muscles strong and joints flexible.
- Use standard precautions when dealing with bleeding.

What should be considered an emergency?

- Call emergency medical services/911 for
  - ~ Head trauma followed by headache, vomiting, change in behavior, or other unusual signs
  - ~ Any bleeding that is not easily stopped after 10 minutes, or any vigorous bleeding
- Call parents/guardians for
  - ~ Swelling of a joint or muscle. Parents/guardians should be notified immediately about any signs or symptoms of bleeding into a muscle or joint such as swelling or inability to move the body part. Older children may recognize the sensation of a joint bleed or notice swelling of their muscle or joint. You should notify parents/guardians immediately.
  - ~ Minor episodes of bleeding that are stopped with first aid.

What types of training or policies are advised?

- First aid for bleeding
- Standard precautions—using gloves, washing hands, and sanitizing surfaces when dealing with blood (See Glossary for further details.)
- Background on hemophilia or von Willebrand disease

What are some related Quick Reference Sheets?

Idiopathic Thrombocytopenic Purpura (page 113)

What are some resources?

- National Hemophilia Foundation, www.hemophilia.org
- National Heart, Lung, and Blood Institute, www.nhlbi. nih.gov/health/dci/Diseases/vWD/vWD_WhatIs.html or http://public.nhlbi.nih.gov/newsroom/home/ GetPressRelease.aspx?id=2553

American Academy of Pediatrics

DEDICATED TO THE HEALTH OF ALL CHILDREN™

Cancer

What is cancer?

- There are many different kinds of childhood cancer.
- The common theme is that cells in the body grow out of control.
- The outlook is good for many types of pediatric cancer, and on average up to 70% of cases of childhood cancer can be cured.
- The cure rate varies depending on the types of cancer, how far it has spread, the age of the child, and other factors. Because of this, many cancer survivors are attending child care and school.
- Children may come to school or child care as cancer survivors, or they may be diagnosed with cancer while enrolled.
- If children who have cancer are well enough during therapy or between rounds of therapy, they may attend child care or school.
- Being with groups of children can provide a routine and the chance to interact with friends, which can be a welcome break from a hospital setting.

How common is it?

- Every year, 14 out of 100,000 children in the United States are diagnosed with some form of cancer.
- The most common cancers are leukemia, lymphoma, and brain cancer.

What are some characteristics of children with cancer?

- Children who are undergoing chemotherapy or radiation to treat their cancer may have a suppressed immune system that can make them more vulnerable to infection.
- Some types of chemotherapy cause hair loss.
- Frequently, children who are receiving cancer therapy will have a central venous catheter in their arm, shoulder, or chest area that provides a way to withdraw blood or give medications without a needlestick. It should be kept dry and protected. The catheter will eventually be removed.

Who is the treatment team?

- Children with cancer are usually treated in special pediatric oncology centers.
- The doctors in those centers are hematologist-oncologists.
- They will manage the child along with the primary care provider in the medical home.
- Because children with cancer may need frequent hospitalizations, often child life specialists in the hospital help children adapt and keep up with any lessons they may miss.

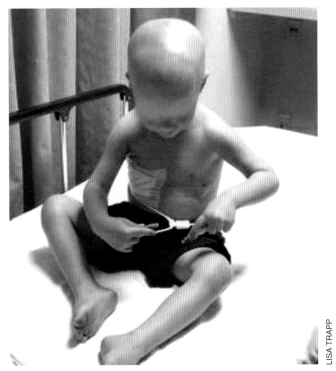

LISA TRAPP

Cancer patient with central line

What adaptations may be needed?

Medications

Some children may be on low-dose antibiotics to prevent infection, but they are usually given at home.

Dietary considerations

There usually is no special diet, but children who are recovering from weight loss from chemotherapy may be on high-calorie foods or shakes.

Physical environment

- Good hygiene such as hand washing and avoiding infectious diseases, especially chickenpox and herpes mouth sores.
- Follow any guidance in the Care Plan about physical activity, but usually children who are well enough to attend child care or school will be able to participate in most activities.
- Develop strategies for accommodating children with cancer. Suggestions include
  ~ Schedule a meeting with parents/guardians to go over the specifics of the particular child's condition because each case is unique.

➤continued

Cancer, continued

~ Have the child make a brief visit before the first full day returning to child care or school to meet with his teachers and classmates.

~ The Care Plan will probably need to be updated frequently for a child who is still getting cancer treatments.

~ Make sure Care Plans are updated after each hospitalization or change in therapy.

~ Explain to the other children about the child's condition, especially if the child's appearance has changed.

~ Children sometimes feel guilty that they somehow caused their condition and may need reassurance that this isn't so.

~ Immediately after chemotherapy or radiation, the child may be more tired or need to rest, but that will resolve over a few weeks.

~ The child may have frequent absences for medical tests and treatments.

What should be considered an emergency?

• Fever is a serious symptom when the child has low blood counts.

• The Care Plan should outline what measures to take if the child has a fever or other symptoms.

What types of training or policies are advised?

Ask the child's oncologist for suggested training resources.

What are some related Quick Reference Sheets?

Altered Immunity: An Overview (page 59)

What are some resources?

• KidsHealth, www.kidshealth.org

• American Cancer Society, www.cancer.org, 800/ACS-2345 (227-2345)

• Starlight Children's Foundation, www.starlight.org

American Academy of Pediatrics

DEDICATED TO THE HEALTH OF ALL CHILDREN™

The information contained in this publication should not be used as a substitute for the medical care and advice of your pediatrician. There may be variations in treatment that your pediatrician may recommend based on individual facts and circumstances.

The American Academy of Pediatrics is an organization of 60,000 primary care pediatricians, pediatric medical subspecialists, and pediatric surgical specialists dedicated to the health, safety, and well-being of infants, children, adolescents, and young adults.

American Academy of Pediatrics
Web site—www.aap.org

Celiac Disease (Gluten-Sensitive Enteropathy)

What is celiac disease?

- Celiac disease, also known as gluten-sensitive enteropathy or sprue, is a digestive disease that results in damage to the small intestine and therefore interferes with the absorption of nutrients from food.
- People who have celiac disease cannot tolerate a protein called gluten, which is found in many foods and everyday products including wheat, rye, and barley.

How common is it?

- Celiac disease affects about 2 million people in the United States, or about 1 in every 133 people. It is often not diagnosed because it is not suspected in individuals.
- Among people who have a first-degree relative with celiac disease, as many as 1 in 22 may have the disease.

What are some characteristics of children with celiac disease?

- Children with celiac disease may have symptoms such as abdominal pain, bloating, diarrhea or constipation, weight loss or weight gain, or unexplained anemia.
- Young children with celiac disease may have poor growth, which begins at the time that they start eating solid foods.
- Children with celiac disease may not have any symptoms, which makes this condition hard to diagnose.
- Other important characteristics include the following:
  ~ Celiac disease is treated by removing all gluten from the diet. The gluten-free diet is a lifetime requirement.
  ~ Without treatment, children with celiac disease can go on to develop anemia, osteoporosis (weak bones), and other complications.
  ~ Children with celiac disease may have a severe itchy, blistering rash known as dermatitis herpetiformis. This rash improves with a gluten-free diet.
  ~ Celiac disease is hereditary, so family members may wish to be tested.

Who is the treatment team?

The treatment team includes a pediatric gastroenterologist and registered dietitians or nutritionists.

What adaptations may be needed?

Medications

- There are no specific medications to treat celiac disease. The proper diet is the main treatment.
- Children who are anemic may be taking iron-supplement medication.

Dietary considerations

- Parents/guardians, caregivers/teachers, and eventually children will need to learn about food selection, label reading, and other strategies to help manage the disease.
- The Care Plan should include lists of "allowed" foods and lists of foods to avoid. In addition, everyone involved in the care of a child with celiac disease should be informed that some other products such as vitamins, stamps, and envelope adhesives contain gluten and should be avoided.
- Ask the child's parents/guardians to provide a list of the child's preferred foods from the "allowed" category.
- Remember that variety is not all that important to young children. They can eat the same thing for lunch every day and be just fine. This may make sticking to a gluten-free diet much easier for these children.
- Ask parents/guardians to suggest or provide a treat for their child to have during classroom celebrations or birthday parties.
- Use the discussion about the child's dietary needs as an opportunity to discuss good nutrition for growing bodies in your classroom.

What should be considered an emergency?

There are no anticipated medical emergencies in celiac disease. In the event of a programmatic emergency, make sure that there is gluten-free food available for the child to eat if necessary.

➤continued

Celiac Disease (Gluten-Sensitive Enteropathy), continued

What are some resources?

- American Dietetic Association, www.eatright.org, 800/877-1600
- Celiac Disease Foundation, www.celiac.org, 818/990-2354
- Gluten Intolerance Group of North America, www.gluten. net, 253/833-6655
- North American Society for Pediatric Gastroenterology, Hepatology and Nutrition, www.naspghan.org
- Gluten-Free Diet Guide for Families, www.cdhnf.org/ user-assets/documents/pdf/GlutenFreeDietGuideWeb.pdf
- The Gluten-free Diet: Some Examples, http://digestive. niddk.nih.gov/ddiseases/pubs/celiac/index.htm#examples

American Academy
of Pediatrics

DEDICATED TO THE HEALTH OF ALL CHILDREN™

Cerebral Palsy

What is cerebral palsy?

- Cerebral palsy, also known as CP, is a condition caused by brain injury that interferes with messages from the brain to the body; this affects movements and muscle coordination.
- The term *cerebral* refers to the brain, and *palsy* means weakness or problems using muscles.

How common is it?

- Each year 8,000 infants and nearly 1,500 preschoolers are diagnosed with CP.
- About 500,000 people in the United States have some form of CP, making this a very common condition.

What are some characteristics of children with cerebral palsy?

- Children may have mild, moderate, or severe CP.
  - ~ Children with *mild* CP may appear to be a little clumsy and have specific difficulties with arm or leg muscle control.
  - ~ Children with *moderate* CP may need adaptive equipment such as leg braces, and may walk with a limp or on their toes.
  - ~ Children with *severe* CP may need a wheelchair or walker to get around.
- There are different types of CP.
  - ~ Children with *spastic* CP, the most common form, have too much muscle tone or tightness. Their legs may come together, for example, when they are picked up, in a manner that is referred to as *scissoring*. They may walk on their toes or in a crouch.
  - ~ Children with *dystonic* CP have difficulty controlling their movements; this causes unusual postures or twisting of their arms or legs that make it hard for them to use their hands or to walk.
  - ~ Children with *mixed* CP have muscles that may be spastic, dystonic, or both. These children may have uncontrolled movements.
- Some children with CP have problems with seeing, hearing, or speaking.
- Children with CP mostly have normal intelligence, but some have intellectual or learning disabilities.
- The muscle problems that children with CP have can often improve with therapy; CP doesn't get worse over time, and most of these children will live as long as their peers.

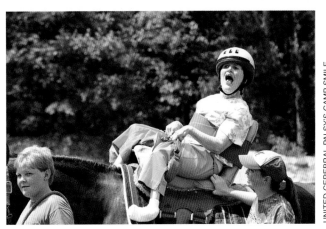

Child with cerebral palsy

UNITED CEREBRAL PALSY'S CAMP SMILE

- Children with CP are more likely to have seizures. If that is the case, see the Seizures, Non-febrile (Epilepsy) Quick Reference Sheet (page 125) for more details.

Who is the treatment team?

- Treatment team members may include the primary care provider, an orthopedist, a pediatric neurologist, and a developmental pediatrician or physical medicine specialist.
- Many children with CP can benefit from different kinds of therapy.
  - ~ *Physical therapy* helps children work on gross-motor skills such as sitting, walking, or balance.
  - ~ *Occupational therapy* helps children develop fine-motor skills necessary for feeding, writing, or dressing.
  - ~ *Speech therapy* is important for children who may need to have the muscles around their face, throat, or tongue strengthened for communication or eating.
- Sometimes medicines or surgery can help lessen the effects of CP.
- Children who are younger than 3 years may receive these therapies through *early intervention* services. Early intervention is a system of services to support infants and toddlers with disabilities and their families.
- For children 3 years and older, *special education and related services* are available through the public schools to provide the therapies necessary for school achievement.

➤*continued*

Cerebral Palsy, continued

What are some elements of a Care Plan for cerebral palsy?

Care Plans may include

- Incorporating physical, speech, or occupational therapy exercises into the child's daily routine. These plans may include the use of splints, braces, communication devices, or adapted toys to help children be more active, participate more, and have fun while they are working their bodies.
- A written plan called the Individualized Family Service Plan will be provided for children in early intervention.
- An Individualized Education Program will describe an older child's unique needs and the services available to address them.

What adaptations may be needed?

Medications

- Some children with CP will have muscle relaxants prescribed.
- Others will get injections done at a specialized treatment center to help relieve muscle spasms.
- If a child with CP has a seizure disorder, she may be taking antiseizure medicines. See the Seizures, Nonfebrile (Epilepsy) Quick Reference Sheet on page 125 for more details.

Dietary considerations

- Children with CP may need a softer or smoother diet if the CP affects their swallowing muscles.
- Depending on the severity of the CP, they also may require extra time and more assistance with meals and snacks than their peers.
- Some children may need a feeding tube.

Physical environment

Develop strategies for accommodating children with cerebral palsy. Suggestions include

- Focus on the individual child and learn firsthand what capabilities and needs he has. Sometimes the physical appearance of a child with CP can give the wrong impression about his ability to learn.

- Remember that despite their physical disabilities, about two thirds of all children with CP have normal intelligence.
- Ask individuals who have cared for children with CP about strategies to help them best learn, and become knowledgeable about different learning styles. Some children will use different techniques such as communication boards to learn.
- Ask the treatment team for tips on how to best adapt lessons and daily routines for the child to develop active learning.
- Work with the physical, occupational, and speech therapists to learn strategies that can best help the child with CP while attending the program or class.

What should be considered an emergency?

- Children with CP may need extra time, supervision, or transport in case of an emergency such as a fire.
- Any critical adaptive equipment would also need to be brought in the event of an evacuation.

What are some resources?

- National Dissemination Center for Children with Disabilities, 800/695-0285 (voice/TTY), www.nichcy.org
- Geralis E. *Children with Cerebral Palsy: A Parent's Guide.* 2nd ed. Bethesda, MD: Woodbine House; 1998
- United Cerebral Palsy, www.ucp.org, 800/872-5827
- Easter Seals, www.easter-seals.org, 800/221-6827

American Academy of Pediatrics

DEDICATED TO THE HEALTH OF ALL CHILDREN™

Cleft Lip and Cleft Palate

What are cleft lip and cleft palate?

- Cleft lip and cleft palate are facial anomalies that are relatively common in newborn babies. A *cleft* is an opening or a separation.
- *Cleft lip* is a separation in the upper lip.
- *Cleft palate* is an opening in the roof of the mouth (known as the *palate*).
- Cleft lip and cleft palate can occur alone or together.

How common are they?

- Cleft lip and cleft palate are among the most common birth defects, affecting more than 5,000 newborns a year in the United States, with an incidence of 1 in 700 newborns.
- Cleft lip and cleft palate can occur alone or in association with known genetic conditions. More than 300 other known genetic conditions have been described in which cleft lip or cleft palate may occur.

What are some characteristics of children with cleft lip or cleft palate?

- The cleft, or opening, in the lip or palate is usually identifiable at the time of birth.
- Less commonly, a cleft occurs only in the muscles of the soft palate but not in the lining of the mouth, so there is no visible opening or separation. This is called a submucous cleft palate and may only be diagnosed after a child has complications, such as difficulty with sucking and feeding, nasal regurgitation of milk, recurrent ear infections, or speech disorders.
- Children with cleft lip, with or without cleft palate, can face a variety of complications related to the defect, including
  - **Feeding.** Babies with cleft palate, and occasionally those with an isolated cleft lip, often have difficulties latching onto the breast or bottle nipple and sucking. This can cause nasal regurgitation (breast milk or formula that comes out of the nose). Often these babies need special bottles and nipples for successful feeding. Most will swallow a great deal of air and require frequent burping. Rarely, special appliances called *obturators* (a prosthetic device that closes the opening of the cleft) are required.
  - **Ear infections and hearing loss.** The cleft causes disruption of the normal muscle anatomy of the palate. This interferes with the eustachian tube that connects the middle ear to the back of the throat, and the malfunction can allow bacteria into the middle ear. Thus, babies with cleft palate are susceptible to repeated ear

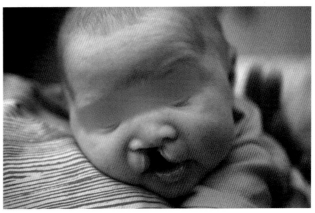

Child with cleft lip

JESS ROLLAR

infections, which over time can cause hearing damage if not treated appropriately.
  - **Dental problems.** If a cleft lip extends through the upper gum and the bone where the teeth are located, the teeth can be missing or abnormal in the area of the cleft.
  - **Speech problems.** The lip and palate are used in forming sounds, so the development of normal speech can be affected. Hearing problems related to fluid that collects in the middle ear and can cause ear infections can affect speech as well.
  - **Psychological problems.** Children with cleft lip and or cleft palate are more likely to have social and emotional problems because of their appearance, speech problems, and related family stress.

Who is the treatment team?

- A treatment team that specializes in the care of children with cleft lip and cleft palate should be involved. The treatment team usually includes the child's primary care provider, a plastic surgeon, a pediatric dentist, a pediatric otolaryngologist (ie, ear, nose, and throat doctor), an audiologist, a speech therapist, and a psychologist or social worker to address family concerns. Other important consultants should include a medical geneticist, an orthodontist, a maxillofacial surgeon, and nurses or occupational therapists who are trained in feeding children with cleft lip or cleft palate.
- Most children with cleft lip will have surgery between birth and 3 months of age to close the lip.
- Cleft palate repair usually occurs by 1 year of age.
- Many children will require follow-up surgeries after age 2.

➤*continued*

Cleft Lip and Cleft Palate, continued

- For children with cleft palate and a collection of fluid in the middle ear or with recurrent ear infections, ear tubes are placed during the palate surgery to prevent ear infections and hearing loss.
- Children who are younger than 3 years may receive speech therapy through local *early intervention* programs. Early intervention is a system of services to support infants and toddlers with disabilities. See Chapter 2 for more details.
- Children 3 years and older may receive speech therapy through *special education and related services* through their local public school system. See Chapter 2 for more details.

What adaptations may be needed?

Dietary considerations

- The Care Plan for an infant with cleft lip or cleft palate may include the use of special feeding devices such as a Haberman Feeder or the Mead Johnson cleft palate nurser (bottles specialized for feeding children with cleft palates) or less frequently, an obturator, which is a special device to close the opening of the cleft.
- For some children with more feeding difficulty, the formula or breast milk may be concentrated or fortified with more calories to help the baby get sufficient calories with lower volumes.
- Feeding a child with a cleft lip or cleft palate should not be rushed but should take no longer than 30 minutes.

Physical environment

Develop strategies for accommodating children with cleft lip or cleft palate. Suggestions include

- Focus on the child as an individual, and point out positive attributes that don't involve physical appearance or speech difficulty.
- Because of potential hearing problems, be aware of the possible need to repeat directions or use visual cues.
- Children with cleft lip or cleft palate may be at risk for teasing by classmates. Be sensitive to this and promote acceptance activities.
- Some children with cleft lip or cleft palate may require additional surgeries, and the child may experience many missed days in child care or school. When the child begins elementary school, it is critical to develop a plan up front to work in partnership with parents/guardians and homebound teachers to ensure that the child's education is ongoing and those transitions go smoothly.

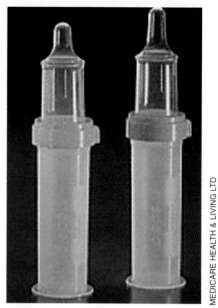

MEDICARE HEALTH & LIVING LTD

The Haberman Feeder is used for children with cleft lips and palates who cannot grip a standard bottle.

- Most children with cleft lip or cleft palate have normal intelligence.
- Work with speech therapists to help children pronounce words clearly.

What should be considered an emergency?

- There are no special emergencies that children with cleft lip or cleft palate face.
- Choking may be a problem in younger children; reviewing first response and first aid training, especially about choking, may be helpful for staff.

What types of training or policies are advised?

- Pediatric first aid training that includes CPR (management of a blocked airway and rescue breathing) with instructional demonstration and return demonstration by participants on a manikin. *Pediatric First Aid for Caregivers and Teachers* is a course designed to teach these skills. Please see "Additional Resources" on page 199 for more information.

What are some resources?

- Cleft Palate Foundation, info@cleftline.org, 919/933-9044
- Children's Craniofacial Association, contactCCA@ccakids.com, 800/535-3643

**American Academy
of Pediatrics**

DEDICATED TO THE HEALTH OF ALL CHILDREN™

The information contained in this publication should not be used as a substitute for the medical care and advice of your pediatrician. There may be variations in treatment that your pediatrician may recommend based on individual facts and circumstances.

The American Academy of Pediatrics is an organization of 60,000 primary care pediatricians, pediatric medical subspecialists, and pediatric surgical specialists dedicated to the health, safety, and well-being of infants, children, adolescents, and young adults.

American Academy of Pediatrics
Web site—www.aap.org

Cystic Fibrosis

What is cystic fibrosis?

- Cystic fibrosis (CF) is an inherited condition that causes mucus and secretions to become thick and sticky. These secretions can then block the lungs, gastrointestinal tract, sinuses, and other parts of the body.
- Children with CF are prone to getting recurrent pneumonias and to having digestive problems because of the mucus blockage of the lungs and digestive system.
- As with most conditions, some children are more severely affected than others.

How common is it?

There are currently about 30,000 children and young adults with CF in the United States.

What are some characteristics of children with cystic fibrosis?

- These children may not appear ill at all, or they may be thin or small.
- They may cough frequently and produce thick mucus. This cough is not contagious like the cough associated with a cold or flu; it is just the body's way of trying to clear mucus.
- Children with CF may have fingertips that are rounded or have a blue tinge.
- Children with CF may require medications and lung treatments, but these medications will not affect attention or ability to learn.
- Some children with CF may have bulky stools or diarrhea and may pass gas more frequently.
- Their skin may taste salty.
- Children with CF need to take pancreatic enzymes before eating and they may need extra vitamins.
- Many places have specialized CF centers; children should get care from a specialist in this disease as well as from their primary care provider.
- Ask the child's parents/guardians who is most involved in their child's care.

Who is the treatment team?

- Children with CF are often cared for in specialized CF centers in addition to their medical home. These centers will often include pediatric pulmonologists, respiratory therapists, nutritionists, and social workers with specific expertise in CF. Other specialists may include gastroenterologists.

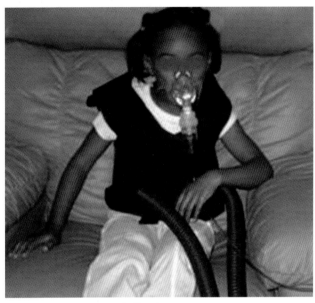

Respiratory therapy for cystic fibrosis

GOLD BAMBOO

What adaptations may be needed?

As always, the Care Plan should be updated after hospitalizations, emergency visits, child absences for illness, and changes in medications.

Medications

- Children with CF are often treated with oral and inhaled antibiotics.
- Nebulized treatments with medications like albuterol may be given to open the airways.
- Other breathing treatments to loosen the mucus are also sometimes given.
- Pancreatic enzymes
  - ~ Store at room temperature in a safe location.
  - ~ Consider allowing older children to carry their own day's supply of enzymes, so they do not have to spend most of their mealtime waiting to get medications instead of eating.
- As always, check the expiration date and develop a system to get new supplies as needed.
- Special vaccines may be necessary, and as for all children, but especially important for those with CF, an annual flu shot is recommended.

➤continued

Cystic Fibrosis, continued

Dietary considerations

- Children with CF should have increased fluids.
- Most of us try to avoid salt and fat, but children with CF may need a little extra salt or fat or to have increased calories.
- Children with CF need to take enzymes before eating. For young children, the enzymes should be opened and sprinkled on a small amount of food.
- Older children will probably swallow capsules directly.
- Ask parents/guardians what foods are best to mix with the enzymes (applesauce is commonly used).

Physical environment

- Special equipment—some children use a special vest for chest physical therapy.
- Caregivers/teachers may want to schedule a visit with parents/guardians to review the specifics of the child's condition. The child may want to make a short visit before coming for a full day, especially after hospitalizations.
- Open bathroom access is important.
- Children with CF should clean their hands frequently and staff should be extra careful about cleaning toys and other children's hands.
- Chest physical therapy helps to clear the mucus out of the airway; children with CF may need chest physical therapy while at child care.
- Children with CF should avoid sharing beverages or foods with other children and other activities that increase the chance of sharing infections because a common cold can turn into pneumonia more easily.
- Absences may occur more often because of hospitalizations and the need to closely monitor minor respiratory illnesses. Help children with CF keep updated with their schoolwork and projects.
- Encourage exercise.
- Children with CF can do almost anything, but may need rest if they tire more easily.

What should be considered an emergency?

- Call emergency medical services/911 for
  - ~ Respiratory distress
  - ~ Sudden chest pain
  - ~ Significant blood in sputum

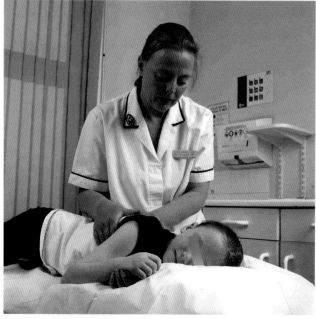

Therapeutic massage opens the lungs in children with cystic fibrosis

CF TRUST

- Call parents/guardians for
  - ~ Fever
  - ~ Change in sputum color or blood streaking
  - ~ Increased fatigue

What types of training or policies are advised?

- Recognizing respiratory emergencies
- Background about CF
- Medication administration

What are some resources?

- Cystic Fibrosis Foundation, www.cff.org, 800/344-4823.
- American Lung Association, www.lungusa.org.
- Local CF centers may be able to hold training sessions or provide materials.

American Academy of Pediatrics

DEDICATED TO THE HEALTH OF ALL CHILDREN™

The information contained in this publication should not be used as a substitute for the medical care and advice of your pediatrician. There may be variations in treatment that your pediatirician may recommend based on individual facts and circumstances.

The American Academy of Pediatrics is an organization of 60,000 primary care pediatricians, pediatric medical subspecialists, and pediatric surgical specialists dedicated to the health, safety, and well-being of infants, children, adolescents, and young adults.

American Academy of Pediatrics
Web site—www.aap.org

Diabetes

What is diabetes?

- Diabetes is a disorder that affects the way the body uses or converts food for energy and growth.
- There are 2 types of diabetes.
  - ~ Type 1 diabetes is a disease in which the immune system destroys the cells in the pancreas that make insulin. Insulin is the hormone that helps our bodies metabolize sugar. Children with type 1 diabetes need to take insulin injections to live.
  - ~ Type 2 diabetes is a condition in which the pancreas produces insulin, but the body cannot use it, often because of obesity; this is known as insulin resistance.
- Both types of diabetes cause glucose, or sugar, to build up in the blood. This glucose can't be used by the body as fuel. The body excretes the excess sugar in the urine, causing increased urination.

How common is it?

- Diabetes affects 20.8 million people in the United States, or about 7% of the population.
- Type 1 diabetes is most common in children, with about 3 million affected. About 1 in 500 US children have type 1 diabetes.
- Type 2 diabetes typically develops in people after age 40, but can be seen earlier. It has recently begun to appear more frequently in children, especially among children who are obese.

What are some characteristics of children with diabetes?

- Symptoms of diabetes can include excessive thirst, frequent urination, increased appetite with weight loss, fatigue, or lethargy. Sudden onset of unexplained wetting (incontinence) is also a warning sign to check for diabetes.
- Children with type 1 diabetes can develop *diabetic ketoacidosis* (DKA), a condition in which their blood glucose is extremely high. A dangerous electrolyte imbalance accompanies the child's high blood glucose. Children in DKA may have vomiting, dehydration, a "fruity" smell to their breath, labored breathing, and progression to unconsciousness and death if not treated.
- Type 2 diabetes generally has a slower and more gradual onset of the same symptoms caused by high sugar levels. Sometimes type 2 diabetes has no symptoms in children and adults.

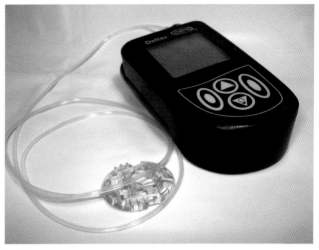
Insulin pump

AAP

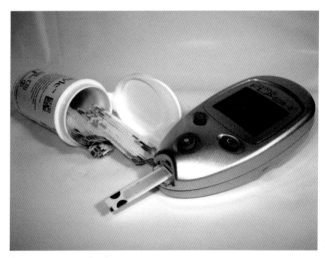
Glucose meter and strips

AAP

- Short-term complications of diabetes are related to blood sugars being too high or too low.
- Long-term complications include vision problems, early heart disease, poor wound healing, high blood pressure, nerve damage, and kidney failure.
- Children with diabetes need exercise and a healthy diet as part of their treatment. They should be given the same opportunities to participate in child care and school activities but may need some adjustment of their insulin or food to accommodate changes in activity.

➤*continued*

Who is the treatment team?

• A pediatric endocrinologist and dietitian often direct the medical management of children with diabetes in association with diabetes nurse educators.

• Often, but not always, there are social workers or psychologists working with such multidisciplinary teams. These professionals may serve as a resource for information or training for your program.

What are some elements of a Care Plan for diabetes?

• All children with diabetes should have an individualized health Care Plan in place before the start of the school year or prior to entrance into child care.

• Following are components of a plan for type 1 diabetes.

~ Managing diabetes requires frequent finger-stick blood tests (to check for blood glucose levels), diet adjustments, and insulin injections. Most children with type 1 diabetes receive their insulin by injections. Some others use a mechanical insulin pump with a plastic catheter placed under their skin.

~ The Care Plan should include

❖ When finger sticks should be checked and how the testing material should be disposed of safely.

❖ What blood sugar range is expected for the child and what actions should be taken immediately if the blood sugar is abnormally high or low.

❖ Where and how insulin injections are given. Ideally there should be a written plan to describe how to adjust insulin doses, how to recognize and treat low blood sugars, and when to call for parental or diabetes-team assistance.

❖ What are typical symptoms of hyperglycemia (blood sugar too high) or hypoglycemia (blood sugar too low) for this child.

❖ The type, frequency, and amount of insulin used. Insulin comes in long- and short-acting varieties that are frequently used together. During the day, most children require only premeal or pre-snack doses of the fast-acting insulin.

❖ Be sure all staff who will care for the child go over the Care Plan with the child's parents/guardians, and keep foods that will correct low blood glucose levels available at all times (eg, juice, glucose tablets or gels).

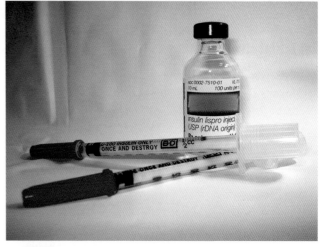

Insulin vial

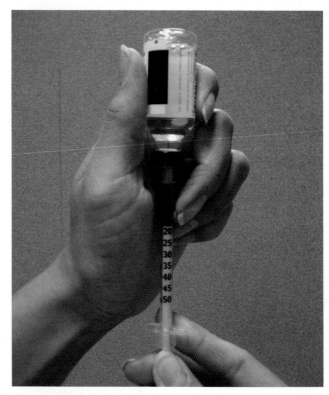

Measuring insulin

❖ Close communication with parents/guardians is essential. The program staff or school nurse should keep a log of the child's blood glucose levels and ask parents/guardians to keep the program informed of blood sugars at home. Parents/guardians should be able to provide logbooks and can work with the program staff to develop a successful communication process.

➤continued

Diabetes, continued

❖ There should be a written plan concerning how to respond to a low or high blood glucose level, and how to reach parents and the pediatric diabetes team for further advice or assistance.

What adaptations may be needed?

Medications

- Children with type 1 diabetes receive insulin injections to control the disorder. More detailed information is listed under "What are some elements of a Care Plan for diabetes?" on the previous page.
- Children with type 2 diabetes are usually on oral medications to control their blood sugar, but sometimes also receive insulin.
- Glucagon is an emergency medication, usually given by injection, that can raise the blood glucose level in an emergency when the child has a critically low glucose level.

Dietary considerations

- Talk to parents/guardians or a registered dietitian/ nutritionist to help plan the child's meals. A written copy of the child's meal plan should be available so that the entire staff is aware of the child's food and snack needs.
- Have parents suggest or supply foods for their child that can be given during class celebrations or birthdays. Be creative about using activities as rewards rather than sweets for all children but especially for the child with diabetes.
- Children with type 2 diabetes are often overweight and may be on a special lower calorie diet.
- Develop strategies for accommodating children with diabetes. Suggestions include
  ~ Learn about the symptoms of low blood sugar and high blood sugar in children, and know what to do about these symptoms.
  ~ Know what causes low blood sugar. A child may develop low blood sugar if a meal or snack is delayed, if her physical activity is higher than normal, or if she does not eat enough food to match the insulin given. Hypoglycemia is rarely seen in Type 2 diabetes.
    ❖ Symptoms of low blood sugar include hunger, shakiness, confusion, vomiting, headache, irritability, or sleepiness.

❖ Severe low blood sugar (hypoglycemia) can occur if such symptoms are undetected and might cause loss of consciousness or seizures. Severe hypoglycemia is a medical emergency and requires glucagon injection and specialty medical assistance. Most low blood sugar levels can be avoided by frequent blood glucose monitoring and awareness of the early signs and symptoms of hypoglycemia by the adults caring for these children.
❖ Orange juice, granulated sugar, jam, or jelly can be given to quickly raise the child's blood sugar.
❖ Glucagon emergency injections are also available for treatment of severe low blood sugar (hypoglycemia) if the child is unable to drink or eat.

~ Know what causes high blood sugar. A child may develop high blood sugar if he is ill or extremely emotionally upset, has not been active, has missed an insulin injection, or has eaten too much food of any kind but especially too many carbohydrates.
  ❖ Symptoms of high blood sugar include frequent urination, thirst, and stomachache.
  ❖ If you suspect high blood sugar, you should check blood glucose levels with a finger stick. If levels are high, drinking water or sugar-free liquid may help. Check the child's Care Plan for other details about interventions such as additional insulin.

Physical environment

Physical activity is important to the health of children with type 2 diabetes, so outdoor play is part of their therapy. Children with type 1 diabetes should be able to play normally. Staff should take a portable pack with insulin, syringes, high-calorie supplements, and glucagon in case of emergency whenever the child is in a different location or on a field trip. A glucometer to check blood sugar should also be available.

What should be considered an emergency?

- Call emergency medical services/911 if the child
  ~ Vomits repeatedly and becomes disoriented or unconscious.

➤continued

Diabetes, continued

  ~ Cannot keep any food or fluids down when his blood sugar is low.
  ~ Develops lethargy or has a seizure.
- Call the parents/guardians or the diabetes team for
  ~ High blood glucose
  ~ Low blood glucose if the child is alert and taking food
  ~ More frequent urination
- In the event of a programmatic emergency needing evacuation, the child's insulin and any necessary emergency equipment must be brought with the child.

What types of training or policies are advised?

- Medication administration
- Dietary guidelines
- Diabetes education for all staff
- Emergency management
- Standard precautions (eg, gloves, hand washing)
- Glucose monitoring

What are some resources?

- Juvenile Diabetes Research Foundation International, 800/533-CURE (533-2873), www.jdrf.org
- The National Diabetes Education Program school guide, *Helping the Student with Diabetes Succeed: A Guide for School Personnel* (free), http://ndep.nih.gov/media/Youth_NDEPSchoolGuide.pdf
- Children With Diabetes online community, www.childrenwithdiabetes.com
- American Diabetes Association, www.diabetes.org
- International Society for Pediatric and Adolescent Diabetes, www.ispad.org

American Academy of Pediatrics

DEDICATED TO THE HEALTH OF ALL CHILDREN™

Down Syndrome

What is Down syndrome?

Down syndrome is a relatively common birth defect caused by extra genetic material from chromosome 21 (ie, there are 3 copies of chromosome 21 rather than 2). This syndrome affects the physical and intellectual development of the child.

How common is it?

- About 4,000 children with Down syndrome are born each year.
- Women of any age can have a baby with Down syndrome, but the risk increases in women older than 35 years.

What are some characteristics of children with Down syndrome?

- Down syndrome causes intellectual disabilities and characteristic facial and physical features, and can be associated with internal malformations.
- All children are different and will have various levels of ability.
- The degree of intellectual disability can be mild, moderate, or severe.
- Medical complications may include heart defects, hearing loss, frequent ear infections, sleep apnea, thyroid disease, and eye disease including cataracts.
- Other rare complications include leukemia, intestinal blockage (atresia), seizures, and hip dislocation.
- A condition called atlantoaxial instability, where the neck bones can slide and cause spinal cord compression, is a risk.
- Children with Down syndrome
  ~ Tend to be short.
  ~ Tend to have low muscle tone.
  ~ May become overweight.
  ~ May be more prone to dental and gum disease.
  ~ May be more susceptible to respiratory infections (colds).
  ~ May get more complications from colds.

Who is the treatment team?

- Children with Down syndrome frequently receive services from early intervention or special child health services for physical, occupational, or speech therapy. See Chapter 2 for more details.

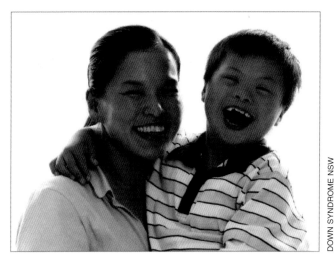

Child with Down syndrome

DOWN SYNDROME NSW

- Children who are younger than 3 years may receive therapies through *early intervention* services. Early intervention is a system of services to support infants and toddlers with disabilities and their families.
- For children 3 years and older, *special education and related services* are available through the public school to provide the accommodations necessary for school achievement.
- Children with Down syndrome will have a primary care provider in their medical home and may have subspecialists involved in their care if they have other specific medical conditions (eg, a pediatric cardiologist for a congenital heart problem).

What adaptations may be needed?

Medications

- Children with Down syndrome do not need specific medications for their syndrome, but they may take medications for an associated condition.
- Children with heart defects may take a diuretic to reduce fluid in their body or a medication to make the heart contract better.
- Children with thyroid disease may take medication to control their condition.
- Annual flu vaccine is recommended for all children and can be especially important for children with Down syndrome who have associated conditions.

➤*continued*

Down Syndrome, continued

Dietary considerations

A special diet may be recommended if medical complications such as obesity or heart conditions are present.

Physical environment

- Special equipment
  - ~ Children with Down syndrome who have hearing loss may need to wear hearing aids. (See page 96 for adaptations for Hearing Loss and Deafness.)
  - ~ Children with eye disease may need glasses or eye patches. (See page 140 for adaptations for Visual Impairments.)
- Develop strategies for accommodating children with Down syndrome. Suggestions include
  - ~ Children with poor muscle tone, coordination challenges, or limited mobility may need additional help, special exercises, or customized activities.
  - ~ Because of the risk of atlantoaxial instability, activities with extreme neck flexion such as somersaults should be avoided. The benefit of doing special radiographs to help determine the risk of neck problems is controversial.
  - ~ Early intervention services such as physical, occupational, or speech therapy may be required and can often be incorporated into other program activities.
  - ~ Other children may need help in understanding the differences in these students.
  - ~ Children with Down syndrome often have good social skills and can serve as a model for other children.
  - ~ Placement of the child in a class depending on age and developmental capabilities may need to be discussed with parents/guardians.

What should be considered an emergency?

- No special medical emergencies are expected in children with Down syndrome other than those associated with medical complications such as congenital heart defects.
- In general emergency situations such as an evacuation for fire, children with Down syndrome may take extra preparation, time, and supervision.

What types of training or policies are advised?

- Caregivers/teachers may need training on how to adapt daily lessons and schedules to accommodate these children.
- Medication administration training may be needed.
- Specific training about the individual child's special needs may be necessary.
- The child's schedule may need to be adapted if individual therapy (ie, physical, occupational, speech) will take place at the program.

What are some resources?

- National Down Syndrome Congress, www.ndsccenter.org, 800/232-6372
- National Down Syndrome Society, www.ndss.org, 800/221-4602
- The Arc, www.thearc.org, 301/565-3842

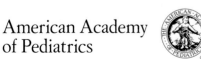

American Academy
of Pediatrics

DEDICATED TO THE HEALTH OF ALL CHILDREN™

The information contained in this publication should not be used as a substitute for the medical care and advice of your pediatrician. There may be variations in treatment that your pediatirician may recommend based on individual facts and circumstances.

The American Academy of Pediatrics is an organization of 60,000 primary care pediatricians, pediatric medical subspecialists, and pediatric surgical specialists dedicated to the health, safety, and well-being of infants, children, adolescents, and young adults.

American Academy of Pediatrics
Web site—www.aap.org

Gastroesophageal Reflux Disease (GERD)

What is gastroesophageal reflux disease (GERD)?

- Gastroesophageal reflux (GER) is a condition in which stomach contents go up into the esophagus (the tube that connects the mouth to the stomach). This occurs commonly in babies and tends to improve as the infant gets older, but sometimes it is severe or does not improve with time.
- When GER causes symptoms in babies other than spitting up, it is called gastroesophageal reflux disease (GERD). Worrisome symptoms include
  - ~ Forceful vomiting
  - ~ Vomiting blood or green-tinged bile
  - ~ Excessive irritability with feeds
  - ~ Breathing problems associated with feeding
  - ~ Failure to gain weight
  - ~ Recurrent pneumonias or asthmas not responding to medications

How common is it?

- Spitting up is very common in infants, but most infants do not have complications and will outgrow the condition quickly.
- When the symptoms do not improve over time and become a problem, it is considered to be a disease. It is difficult to estimate how many children have the official diagnosis of GERD.

What are some characteristics of children with GERD?

- Symptoms of GERD could include abdominal or chest pain, breathing problems, irritability, unexplained anemia, difficulty swallowing, or hoarse voice, especially in the morning.
- In older children and adults, these symptoms prompt people to seek medical attention and by definition they have GERD.
- Gastroesophageal reflux disease peaks at 2 to 4 months of age and usually starts improving at 6 to 12 months of age as the child learns to sit alone. Sometimes older children and adults have GERD as well. Older children may be able to mention these symptoms, but babies cannot express them.
- Babies tend to have symptoms such as back arching, irritability, spitting up, nasal congestion, and cough or wheezing. Some babies can even stop breathing (apnea) or have a slow heart rate because of GERD.

What adaptations may be needed?

Medications

- Different kinds of medications may be used to block the stomach acid from causing irritation to the esophagus (food pipe).
- Some medications block the production of stomach acids.
- Some of these are available over the counter (OTC) and some are prescribed. The child's primary care provider or specialist (eg, pediatric gastroenterologist) should be supervising any of these treatments in babies or young children.
- Antacids neutralize stomach acid. Most of these are available OTC. These medications usually have no serious side effects.

Dietary considerations

- To keep the stomach from being full and triggering the backflow of food, feeding smaller meals on a 3-hour schedule can help.
- Some people find that thickening a baby's formula or expressed breast milk with rice cereal helps. Sometimes the nipple will need to be enlarged a little to allow the flow of the formula, but it shouldn't be wide enough to allow the baby to gulp the formula too quickly.

Physical environment

- Upright positioning on a slope that does not increase pressure on the abdomen for 30 to 60 minutes after feedings; burping before, halfway through, and after the meal; and avoiding tight diapers can help infants with GERD.
- Research shows that all babies, including those with GERD, are safer if they sleep on their backs. They should never be placed to sleep on their stomachs or sides.
- Older children should avoid clothing that puts pressure on the abdomen and shouldn't lay down for a nap immediately after eating.

What should be considered an emergency?

Babies with GERD can choke; a bulb syringe should be available to help clear the airway if necessary. If the baby is coughing, nothing should be done because the cough is the most effective way to clear the airway. If the baby stops breathing or making any sound, CPR techniques for infants should be used. These maneuvers are covered in pediatric first aid with CPR courses such as the American Academy of Pediatrics course, *Pediatric First Aid for Caregivers and Teachers.*

➤continued

Gastroesophageal Reflux Disease (GERD), continued

What types of training or policies are advised?

- First aid to clear the airway for choking.
- Feeding techniques including upright positioning and frequent burping.
- Nutrition consultation on preparing thickened feeds may be helpful.
- Feeding therapy consultation may be helpful.
- Medication administration if medications are to be given while in care.

What are some resources?

Caring for Our Children: National Health and Safety Performance Standards: Guidelines for Out-of-Home Child Care Programs, 2nd Edition, standards 4.007, 4.009, and 4.011 through 4.021

American Academy
of Pediatrics

DEDICATED TO THE HEALTH OF ALL CHILDREN™

Gastrostomy Tubes

What are gastrostomy tubes?

- A gastrostomy tube, or G-tube, is a small tube placed directly into a child's stomach for the purpose of providing food, fluid, or medicines without having to go through the mouth.
- Gastrostomy tubes appear like a small cap on the outside of a child's stomach.

How common are they?

Gastrostomy tubes are placed in children for many reasons, including prematurity, feeding problems, and brain disorders, and they have become more prevalent as lifesaving medical treatments for children have improved.

Who is the treatment team?

- A child with a G-tube may be under the care of a pediatric gastroenterologist or surgeon.
- Often a nurse or dietitian is available at the specialist's office to answer questions related to the G-tube.

What are some elements of a Care Plan for gastrostomy tubes?

The child's Care Plan will include flushing, giving feedings and medications, and venting the tube.

1. **Flushing the G-tube**
   ~ It is important to flush the G-tube before and after any tube feedings, before and after any medications, or at least every 8 hours. Flushing involves putting water in a syringe and injecting it into the G-tube.
2. **To give feedings through a G-tube, you will need**
   ~ Catheter-tip syringe (35 or 60 mL)
   ~ Formula
   ~ Measuring cup
   ~ Extension set, if desired
   ~ Procedure
     1. Explain the procedure to the child.
     2. Wash your hands with soap and water.
     3. Assemble all the supplies.
     4. Pour the correct amount of formula into a clean measuring cup or clean baby bottle.
     5. Place the child in a comfortable position. If possible, place the child in a high chair at the table during mealtimes.
     6. Insert the syringe tip into the feeding tube.

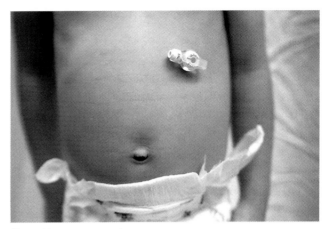
Child with gastrostomy tube

AAP

7. Flush tubing with 3 to 5 mL of water or as directed by the child's health care professional prior to starting the formula feeding.
8. Slowly pour the formula into the syringe.
9. Unclamp the feeding tube. The feeding rate can be controlled by raising or lowering the syringe. The feeding should take about the same amount of time as it would take a child to drink the formula—about 15 to 20 minutes. Stop the feeding if the child becomes nauseated, shows signs of abdominal discomfort, is vomiting, or has difficulty breathing.
10. If the child cannot be fed by mouth, oral stimulation with a pacifier can be provided during the gastrostomy feeding.
11. When all the formula has been given, flush the tubing with water as directed by the child's health care professional, recap the tube or disconnect all tubing, and close the cap on the G-tube button.
12. Try burping the child after each feeding if appropriate.
13. Medicines can be pushed directly into the G-tube through a syringe.
14. Rinse the feeding supplies with warm water after each feeding and allow to air-dry. Replace syringes and extension sets every 2 weeks.

~ If the formula is backing up, try
   ❖ Changing the position of the tubing to slow the rate
   ❖ Changing the child's position
   ❖ Flushing the feeding tube with 3 to 5 mL of tap water

3. **Venting the tube**
   ~ You may need to vent the child's tube to remove excess air or fluid in the child's stomach.

➤continued

Gastrostomy Tubes, continued

~ Open the G-tube port and attach to a drainage device (eg, mucous trap, drainage bag). You may be asked to measure and record the amount of drainage.

What adaptations may be needed?

Dietary considerations

- Children in school or child care who have G-tubes often will require feedings or medications through the tube.
- Discuss ways to develop the child's oral motor skills if the G-tube is for feeding problems. Often, using a pacifier during feedings promotes oral motor skills.

Physical environment

- Staff should be trained in how to open a G-tube so that extra gas in the stomach can escape (see "3. Venting the tube" in the Care Plan procedure).
- Do not allow the child to pull on the tube. A one-piece, snap T-shirt works best for infants and toddlers. Keep the tube secured beneath the child's clothing.
- It is important to know what size and type tube the child has.
- Designate at least one caregiver/teacher per shift as the G-tube captain. Plan an in-service for all staff to promote comfort with this device.

What should be considered an emergency?

- Call emergency medical services/911 if
  - ~ The child's stomach is hard and bloated, and you cannot vent the G-tube.
  - ~ The child develops forceful vomiting.
- Notify parents/guardians if
  - ~ The G-tube is pulled out. You can cover the area with a small, clean dressing and tape. The tube needs to be replaced within 4 hours.
  - ~ You notice redness, irritation, or foul odor around the stomach.
  - ~ The G-tube is leaking.
  - ~ Skin or excess tissue seems to be growing around the tube opening.
  - ~ The G-tube is clogged and flushing does not help.

What types of training or policies are advised?

- Medical administration
- Tube feeding
- Standard precautions

What are some resources?

- Cincinnati Children's Hospital Medical Center, 513/636-4200, 800/344-2462, 513/636-4900 (TTY)
- New York State Department of Health Emergency Medical Services, www.health.state.ny.us/nysdoh/ems/pdf/referencecard.pdf

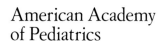

American Academy
of Pediatrics

DEDICATED TO THE HEALTH OF ALL CHILDREN™

The information contained in this publication should not be used as a substitute for the medical care and advice of your pediatrician. There may be variations in treatment that your pediatrician may recommend based on individual facts and circumstances.

The American Academy of Pediatrics is an organization of 60,000 primary care pediatricians, pediatric medical subspecialists, and pediatric surgical specialists dedicated to the health, safety, and well-being of infants, children, adolescents, and young adults.

American Academy of Pediatrics
Web site—www.aap.org

Hearing Loss and Deafness

What are hearing loss and deafness?

- The terms *hearing loss* and *hard of hearing* describe a wide range of conditions that partially or totally prevent individuals from receiving sound in all or most of its forms.
- Children with hearing loss may hear sounds very differently. Some children respond well to hearing amplification, such as hearing aids, and can hear speech clearly. Other children may have very little response to sounds in their environment.
- New technology such as cochlear implants can affect the quality of a child's hearing.
- The Individuals With Disabilities Education Act (IDEA) includes "hearing impairment" and "deafness" as 2 separate categories under which children may be eligible for special education and related services programming.
  - ~ Hearing loss is defined by IDEA as "an impairment in hearing, whether permanent or fluctuating, that adversely affects a child's educational performance."
  - ~ Deafness is defined as "a hearing loss that is so severe that the child is impaired in processing linguistic information through hearing, with or without amplification."

How common are they?

- Hearing loss affects individuals of all ages and may occur at any time from infancy through adulthood. Current US Department of Education statistics mention that 1.3% of all students with disabilities receive special education services under the category of "hearing impairment."
- Information from the universal newborn hearing screening literature suggests that 1 to 3 children per 1,000 are identified with hearing loss now that all newborns are screened. Other statistics suggest that 6 per 1,000 school-aged children have hearing loss.
- Mild hearing loss is only diagnosed after it is suspected because the screening equipment does not screen for mild hearing loss.

What are some characteristics of children with hearing loss or deafness?

- Children with hearing loss may have difficulty with sensing the loudness or intensity of sound (measured in units called decibels, dB), or the frequency or pitch of sound (measured in units called hertz, Hz).

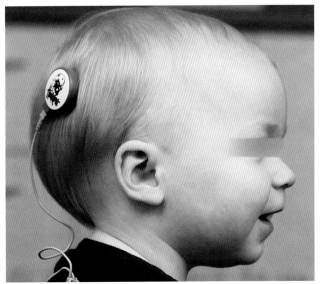

Child with cochlear implant

BOYS TOWN NATIONAL RESEARCH HOSPITAL

- Hearing loss is generally described as *slight, mild, moderate, severe,* or *profound.* The severity of hearing loss depends on how well a person can hear the intensities or frequencies most greatly associated with speech.
- Children whose hearing loss is greater than 90 dB are considered deaf for the purposes of educational placement.
- There is increasing awareness that children with mild or unilateral hearing loss have difficulties in certain settings, especially in noisy environments.
- There are 4 types of hearing loss.
  - ~ *Conductive* hearing loss occurs when diseases of the outer or middle ear cause an obstruction of the pathway of sound to reach the inner ear. Middle ear fluid from chronic ear infections can cause this type of hearing loss. Conductive hearing loss can be helped by hearing aids or surgery.
  - ~ *Sensorineural* hearing loss results from damage to the delicate sensory hair cells of the inner ear or surrounding nerves. Children with this type of hearing loss may hear certain frequencies better than others. Sensorineural hearing loss may perceive distorted sounds with hearing aids, making this condition more difficult to treat.
  - ~ *Mixed* hearing loss refers to a combination of conductive and sensorineural hearing loss. These children may have problems with the outer/middle ear and the inner ear. They may do well with hearing aids, but may experience difficulty during a cold or an ear infection.

➤*continued*

~ *Central* hearing loss results from damage to the nerves of the central nervous system, either in the pathways to the brain or in the brain itself.

Who is the treatment team?

- The treatment team for children with hearing loss includes the pediatrician or primary care provider, pediatric otolaryngologists, audiologists, speech therapists, and education specialists.
- Pediatricians and other primary care providers are important in the management of ear infections, which often lead to more impairment for these children.
- A young child with hearing loss is at high risk of having receptive and expressive language difficulties, so *early intervention* is necessary. Early intervention is a system of services to support infants and toddlers with disabilities and their families. These therapists can work with caregivers/teachers to incorporate exercises and equipment into the day-to-day lives of the children.
- For children 3 years and older, *special education and related services* are available through the public school to provide therapies necessary for school achievement.

What are some elements of a Care Plan for hearing loss and deafness?

The Care Plan for children with hearing loss may include
- Regular speech, language, and auditory training (if chosen by a family)
- Amplification systems such as hearing aids, FM systems, and cochlear implants
- Interpreter services for those children who use sign language
- Preferential seating in class to facilitate lip reading
- Captioned films, videos, and DVDs
- Assistance of a note taker for students with hearing loss so that they may fully attend to instruction
- Alternative communication methods and devices
- Counseling

What adaptations may be needed?

Medications

Children with cochlear implants may be at increased risk of acquiring bacterial meningitis, and these children should refer to their health professional's specific immunization recommendations related to pneumococcal and *Haemophilus influenzae* type b vaccines.

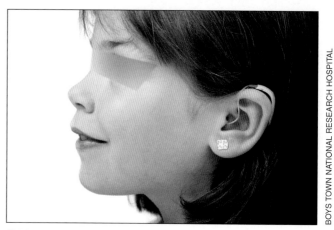

Child with hearing aid

BOYS TOWN NATIONAL RESEARCH HOSPITAL

Physical environment

- Most children with hearing loss are born to hearing parents who have had to learn communication strategies with their child. Partner with parents/guardians to learn how to best communicate with a child who has hearing loss.
- Vocabulary, grammar, word order, and figures of speech may be much more difficult for children with hearing impairments. Early and consistent use of visible communication modes (eg, sign language) is important.
- Children with hearing loss use oral communication (eg, speech, lip reading, residual hearing) or manual communication (eg, signs, finger spelling), or a combination of both (known as total communication) to learn.
- Text telephones (known as TTs, TTYs, or TDDs) enable hearing-impaired students to type phone messages over a telephone network known as the Telecommunications Relay Services. Technologic advances such as video relay, text pagers, and visual fire alarms are available. These can be accessed all over the United States by dialing 711, and the relay service is free.

What should be considered an emergency?

Hearing loss does not lead to any specific emergency situation, although some children with hearing loss may have another condition (eg, seizure disorder) where an emergency medical services (EMS)/911 plan is necessary. In this situation, the EMS/911 plan should include measures to enhance communication with the child during an emergency. Children with hearing loss may need special attention in a programmatic emergency such as a fire.

➤*continued*

Hearing Loss and Deafness, continued

What types of training or policies are advised?

- Sign language—learning some key signs can help with communicating with the child. Other situations call for having a sign language interpreter available.
- In-service from speech therapists or other professionals.

What are some resources?

- National Dissemination Center for Children with Disabilities, 800/695-0285 (voice/TTY), www.nichcy.org
- American Society for Deaf Children, 800/942-2732 (voice/TTY), www.deafchildren.org
- American Speech-Language-Hearing Association, 800/638-8255, 301/296-5650 (TTY), www.asha.org
- Hands & Voices, 303/492-6283, www.handsandvoices.org
- Boys Town National Research Hospital, www.babyhearing.org
- Alexander Graham Bell Association for the Deaf and Hard of Hearing, 202/337-5220, 202/337-5221 (TTY), info@ agbell.org, www.agbell.org

American Academy
of Pediatrics

DEDICATED TO THE HEALTH OF ALL CHILDREN™

Heart Conditions: An Overview

What are heart conditions?

- Children have very different kinds of heart disease than adults. Here is an overview of the categories of heart defects that children have.
  - ~ *Congenital heart defects.* These are structural heart defects that children are born with. They can be very serious and need surgery immediately, or they can be less serious and just need to be watched over time.
  - ~ *Rhythm problems.* The heart can beat too fast, too slow, or too irregularly. This can be an isolated problem or it can be related to other heart disease.
  - ~ *Carditis.* This is a general term for inflammation of the heart. Children can get carditis from viral infections or other diseases such as Kawasaki disease. It can also be called *myocarditis.*
  - ~ *Cardiomyopathy.* This is a term for an abnormal heart muscle. It can be caused by a viral infection or chemical, or it can happen for unknown reasons. Because it can be caused by many different things, it can often be hard to predict how serious it will be or how long it will last. Children may fall anywhere on the spectrum of recovering completely or needing a heart transplant.
  - ~ *Valvular heart disease.* The heart has valves that allow the blood to pass from one area to another. If those valves leak or cause blockage, it can cause heart problems.
- Other important terms
  - ~ *Heart murmur.* A heart murmur is just a sound that the blood makes as it goes through the heart. Often this causes no problems at all. Just like snoring is caused by air going through narrow passages, the blood can be noisy as it travels but pass through without harm. These are called *innocent* or *benign* murmurs. Sometimes a heart murmur is a clue that there is a more serious heart problem.

  - ~ *Cyanosis.* This refers to a blue color of the skin that comes when the blood does not have enough oxygen.
  - ~ *Heart failure.* When the heart fails, it means that it cannot keep up with the workload and it falls behind. It doesn't mean that the heart stops; it just means that it can't pump blood as fast as it needs to.
- For this book, we are going to break heart conditions into 2 groups.
  - ~ *Functional* heart conditions—problems with the functioning of the heart because of infection or other medical issues that develop after birth
  - ~ *Structural* heart defects—problems with the structure of the heart that are usually present at birth
- Children with congenital heart defects can have functional heart conditions caused by the original heart problem, the results of the surgical repair, or their medications.
- Children with congenital heart defects are more likely to enter child care or school with the diagnosis. Functional heart conditions can be present before the child enrolls or can develop while the child is attending the program.
- Sometimes, children with heart problems have other conditions, such as Down, Marfan, or Noonan syndromes. Those other conditions can cause challenges other than the heart problem.

What are some related Quick Reference Sheets?

- Heart Conditions, Functional (page 101)
- Heart Defects, Structural (page 105)

American Academy
of Pediatrics

DEDICATED TO THE HEALTH OF ALL CHILDREN™

Heart Conditions, Functional

What are some characteristics of children with functional heart conditions?

- Children with heart conditions may only have problems intermittently or for a short period.
- These children often have pediatric cardiologists helping with their management in addition to a primary care provider in the medical home.
- The children seldom require other special therapists to be involved in their care, but the specifics of the child's situation should be discussed with parents/guardians.
- This Quick Reference Sheet will provide information on
  ~ Kawasaki disease
  ~ Arrhythmia
  ~ Hypertension (high blood pressure)
  ~ Cardiomyopathy

Kawasaki Disease

What is Kawasaki disease?

- Kawasaki disease is a condition in which the blood vessels become inflamed, especially in the heart where the coronary arteries supply blood to the heart muscle.
- Children with early Kawasaki disease usually have high fever, red eyes, and swollen hands and lips that become cracked as they heal.
- They can also have a rash, swollen mouth and tongue, and swollen lymph nodes.
- This disease is not well understood and its cause is unknown. It can be very tricky to diagnose because there is no test to specifically diagnose the disease.
- Children are usually hospitalized when they have the acute disease, but some of the most serious complications can happen in the recovery stage during the month or two after the disease begins. At that time, the coronary arteries can get weak spots that balloon out and cause aneurysms (see Figure at right).
- Luckily, even though Kawasaki disease is not well understood, it can be treated. Many of the complications can be avoided with treatment and monitoring. Often, children make a complete recovery from Kawasaki disease.

How common is it?

Approximately 4,000 children are diagnosed with Kawasaki disease every year and most are younger than 5 years.

What adaptations may be needed?

Medications

- Children recovering from Kawasaki disease may need to take low-dose aspirin for awhile until it is certain that they have recovered completely.
  ~ The aspirin may cause stomach irritation.
  ~ Parents/guardians should be notified immediately if there is blood when the child has a bowel movement or vomits.
  ~ Aspirin is given to prevent blood clots, so the child might bruise more easily or bleed more if cut.

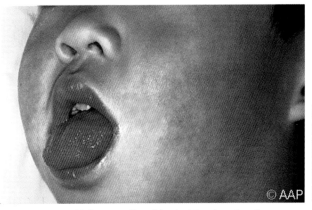

Child with Kawasaki disease with striking facial rash and erythema of the oral mucous membrane

AAP RED BOOK® ONLINE

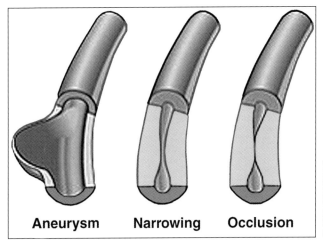

Aneurysm **Narrowing** **Occlusion**

CLEVELAND CLINIC

Kawasaki disease can cause aneurysms to form in blood vessels.

➤continued

- Children recovering from Kawasaki disease should avoid children with chickenpox or the flu if they are on aspirin because of the risk of Reye syndrome, a serious illness that causes liver and brain dysfunction. All children should be vaccinated against chickenpox and influenza, but this is especially important for children who are on aspirin therapy.
- Vaccination—the medication used to treat Kawasaki disease in the hospital, called gamma or immune globulin, can interfere with the effectiveness of live vaccines like measles, mumps, rubella (MMR), and varicella (chickenpox), and those vaccines may need to be delayed for a period. The children should have a note from their primary care provider and should be vaccinated by 1 year after administration of the immune globulin.

Dietary considerations

Usually no special diet is needed.

Physical environment

Most children with Kawasaki disease usually recover completely and need no special adaptations.

What should be considered an emergency?

Seldom a problem, but if the child has a complication, it may present as chest pain or paleness.

What are some resources?

- American Heart Association, www.americanheart.org
- Kawasaki Disease Foundation, www.kdfoundation.org, 978/356-2070

Arrhythmia

What is arrhythmia?

- Arrhythmia is an irregular heartbeat. The heart normally sends a regular electrical signal that makes the heart muscle contract in a proper order. If that signal order is not working well, the heart can have an irregular beat.
- This disorder may interfere with the heart's ability to pump blood.
- The feelings that it causes are called *heart palpitations;* they can be difficult sensations for a child to describe.
- Many people have experienced minor palpitations that are usually not serious. They can be caused by stress or substances like caffeine or cold medications.
- Some forms of arrhythmia are very serious and need immediate treatment. Some of the more serious types of arrhythmias can be caused by conditions such as prolonged QT interval, cardiomyopathy, or Wolf-Parkinson-White syndrome.

- Children who have congenital heart disease may have arrhythmias.
- Arrhythmias that occur in the top chambers of the heart are called *atrial,* such as atrial fibrillation or flutter.
- Arrhythmias that occur in the bottom heart chambers are called ventricular, such as *ventricular* tachycardia.
- These conditions may be treated with medication, surgical procedures on the heart's electrical conduction system, or pacemakers.

What adaptations may be needed?

Medications

- A number of different medications may be prescribed to prevent an irregular heartbeat. Ask the child's parents/guardians and doctors to explain the medications and their side effects.
- Avoid over-the-counter medications unless specifically approved by the child's doctor.

Dietary considerations

Avoid caffeine-containing food or drinks such as coffee, tea, or chocolate unless approved by the child's doctor.

Physical environment

- Because there are many different types and causes of arrhythmia, it is important to customize the child's Care Plan to match the specific situation.
- Activity—usually unrestricted but the child should be allowed to rest if needed.
- Some arrhythmias require restriction of certain athletic activities in schools.

What should be considered an emergency?

- Symptoms like paleness, sweating, dizziness, fainting, chest pain, or shortness of breath may be serious.
- Learn to monitor a pulse.
- Call emergency medical services/911 immediately if the child is having serious symptoms.

What types of training or policies are advised?

- Pediatric first aid training that includes CPR (management of a blocked airway and rescue breathing) with instructional demonstration and return demonstration by participants on a manikin. *Pediatric First Aid for Caregivers and Teachers* is a course designed to teach these skills.
- If there is a child with an arrhythmia enrolled, it is important to have a responsible caregiver who can competently provide CPR on site at all times.
- A CPR-trained person should be available during transport to and from the program if applicable.

➤continued

Heart Conditions, Functional, continued

Hypertension (High Blood Pressure)

What is hypertension (high blood pressure)?

- Hypertension is much less common in children than adults.
- High blood pressure in younger children usually has another cause such as a kidney problem or other medical condition. (See Kidney/Urinary Problems on page 115 for further details.)
- Older children may develop *essential hypertension,* which is high blood pressure without a known cause, especially if they have a strong family history.

What adaptations may be needed?

Medications

Avoid over-the-counter medications unless specifically approved by the child's doctor.

Dietary considerations

- Children with high blood pressure may be on a low-salt diet.
- Children should avoid products that contain caffeine such as chocolate, tea, or coffee.

Physical environment

If a child in the child care center or school has hypertension, ask the parent/guardian to get information specific for that child.

Cardiomyopathy

What is cardiomyopathy?

- Cardiomyopathy is the name for diseases of the heart muscle. It can have many different causes and different outcomes depending on the cause.
- Children with cardiomyopathy are at increased risk for arrhythmias, heart failure, and sudden death.

How common is it?

There are about 1,000 to 5,000 new cases per year in the United States.

What adaptations may be needed?

Physical environment

Cardiomyopathy is relatively uncommon, but it is a condition that should be discussed at length with parents/guardians and the child's doctor.

What types of training or policies are advised?

- How to take a pulse
- Emergency situations/CPR

What are some resources?

- American Heart Association, www.americanheart.org
- Congenital Heart Information Network, http://tchin.org, 609/822-1572

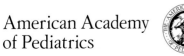

American Academy
of Pediatrics

DEDICATED TO THE HEALTH OF ALL CHILDREN™

The information contained in this publication should not be used as a substitute for the medical care and advice of your pediatrician. There may be variations in treatment that your pediatirician may recommend based on individual facts and circumstances.

The American Academy of Pediatrics is an organization of 60,000 primary care pediatricians, pediatric medical subspecialists, and pediatric surgical specialists dedicated to the health, safety, and well-being of infants, children, adolescents, and young adults.

American Academy of Pediatrics
Web site — www.aap.org

Heart Defects, Structural

What are structural heart defects?

- Cyanotic congenital heart defects
  - ~ Cyanotic defects are very serious and cause the baby to have very low oxygen levels shortly after birth.
  - ~ Examples of cyanotic heart defects are transposition of the great vessels, tetralogy of Fallot, or hypoplastic left heart.
  - ~ These babies usually have heart surgery early in life and often have multiple heart surgeries to correct the defects.
- There are other congenital heart defects of different types. Some make the heart work too hard because it has to pump blood against a blockage, and some increase the amount of blood the heart has to pump.
- Some congenital heart defects need surgery; some need medications; some need no special treatment.
- Some babies with congenital heart disease might need surgery but may be able to wait awhile to grow first. Examples of these are ventricular septal defect (VSD), atrial septal defect, or patent ductus arteriosis. Valve problems like pulmonic or aortic stenosis can also fall in this category.
- Some babies have subtle heart defects that might not be diagnosed for years. Sometimes they heal on their own; other times they need to be treated. Small, muscular VSDs can sometimes close spontaneously.
- Some conditions, such as coarctation of the aorta (in which the major blood vessel that supplies the body is narrowed), require treatment but can be missed for years because they don't cause obvious symptoms.

How common are they?

Thirty-five thousand babies are born every year in the United States with these problems, according to the American Heart Association.

What are some characteristics of children with structural heart defects?

If the heart defect is minor or was completely repaired, the baby or child may appear normal or may just have a scar on the chest. If the defect was not fully repaired, the baby or child may have

- Cyanosis, which is a blue color that is most easily seen around the mouth and lips.
- Feeding difficulties, or the baby or child may tire more easily with feedings or exercise. Some babies have difficulty gaining weight.

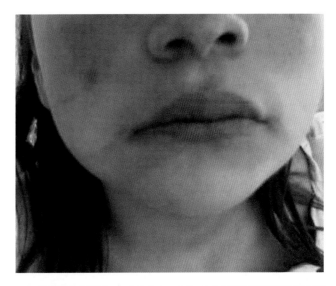
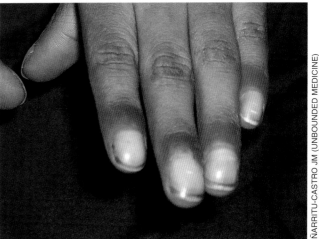

Cyanosis and clubbing in a child with tetralogy of Fallot

IÑARRITU-CASTRO JM (UNBOUNDED MEDICINE)

- Arrhythmias or irregular heartbeat. (See Heart Conditions, Functional on page 101 for more information.)

Who is the treatment team?

- Pediatric cardiac surgery is often performed in special centers that are equipped to handle babies and young children.
- Pediatric cardiologists are involved in the care along with the primary care provider in the medical home.
- Children who have had cardiac surgery may need developmental therapy to help them gain their strength and catch up with the milestones they missed while they were ill or recovering from surgery.
- Speech therapists and nutritionists may help with feeding issues.

➤continued

Heart Defects, Structural, continued

What adaptations may be needed?

Medications

- Many children will not require medication. Those that do will usually have oral medications to
  - ~ Strengthen the heart, like digoxin. This can usually be given at home. Digoxin (Lanoxin is one brand name) must be given very carefully and can cause irregular heartbeats if not dosed correctly.
  - ~ Reduce the fluid in the body with diuretics like furosemide (Lasix). This also will likely be given at home. Diuretics can alter the body's balance of salts and this must be monitored closely. Some children may need extra potassium.
  - ~ Prevent arrhythmias.
- No over-the-counter medications should be given unless approved by the child's doctor.
- Influenza vaccine—all children should get the flu vaccine, but it is especially important for children with heart disease.

Dietary considerations

- Some babies with heart defects may need extra calories to help them to grow.
- They may need small, frequent feedings if they tire easily, and they may feed more slowly than other babies or children in the group.

Physical environment

There are usually few medical restrictions on physical activity, but the child may tire more easily and should be allowed to rest.

What should be considered an emergency?

- Heart defects can vary dramatically and the Care Plan should outline the particular symptoms to watch for in that particular child and how to respond. Some conditions that may be mentioned include
  - ~ Arrhythmia (irregular heart rate)
  - ~ Cyanosis (blue color usually most easily seen around the mouth)
- The Care Plan should outline when to call emergency medical services/911 and when calling parents is sufficient.

What types of training or policies are advised?

- How to check a pulse.
- Pediatric first aid training that includes CPR (management of a blocked airway and rescue breathing) with instructional demonstration and return demonstration by participants on a manikin. *Pediatric First Aid for Caregivers and Teachers* is a course designed to teach these skills.
- It is important if you have a child with a serious arrhythmia to have a responsible caregiver who knows CPR, including cardiac resuscitation, on site at all times.
- If the baby needs special formula or is a slow feeder, training on feeding techniques by a nutritionist or feeding therapist may be helpful.

What are some resources?

Congenital Heart Information Network, http://tchin.org, 609/822-1572

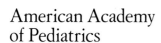

American Academy of Pediatrics

DEDICATED TO THE HEALTH OF ALL CHILDREN™

Hepatitis

What is hepatitis?

- Hepatitis is the name for liver inflammation. The term is usually used for a viral infection of the liver, with hepatitis A, B, or C being the most common. Other viruses like cytomegalovirus (CMV) and Epstein-Barr virus (EBV, also known as infectious mononucleosis or mono) can cause hepatitis. Viral types of hepatitis are contagious, but the risk of spread and how they are spread vary between types. Hepatitis A, EBV, and CMV are transmitted through stool and secretions, but hepatitis B and C are spread by exposure to contaminated blood.
- Hepatitis can also be caused by noninfectious causes such as medications, chemicals, trauma, and certain metabolic diseases. These types of hepatitis are not contagious.
- Hepatitis can be acute (come and go quickly) or chronic (long term). Some children with chronic liver disease will need a liver transplant.

How common is it?

- In the pre-vaccine era, hepatitis A was one of the most commonly reported vaccine-preventable illnesses, with more than 26,000 cases per year reported to the Centers for Disease Control and Prevention. However, since the introduction of a vaccine, incidence of hepatitis A in the United States has declined dramatically, with only 5,683 cases reported in 2004. Previously rates where higher among children than adults, but since institution of the vaccine, rates among children 5 to 14 years of age have been among the lowest.
- Hepatitis B, also a vaccine-preventable infection, may be transmitted vertically from infected mothers to their babies or horizontally through contact with infected blood or sexual contact. Horizontal transmission occurs primarily in adolescents and adults. The recommendation for universal testing of mothers for hepatitis B and universal immunization of children at the time of birth has significantly lowered hepatitis B infection in children. Currently in the United States, 5% to 8% of the total population has been infected, and 0.2% to 0.9% of the population has chronic infection.
- Hepatitis C infection in the United States is estimated at 1.8% of the general population. Currently there is no vaccine against hepatitis C.

What are some characteristics of children with hepatitis?

- Children younger than 6 years usually have few or no signs or symptoms. Symptoms are more common in older children and adults.
- Jaundice, which is a yellow tint of the skin or eyes, is a common symptom.
- Other symptoms may include
  - ~ Chronic itchiness
  - ~ Dark-colored urine or clay-colored stools
  - ~ Poor appetite, nausea or vomiting, and stomach pain
  - ~ Less energy, sleeping more, and having a low-grade fever

Who is the treatment team?

- The primary care provider in the medical home.
- Pediatric gastroenterologists may be involved.
- Pediatric infectious disease specialists may be involved.
- Parents/guardians do not have to share information about hepatitis with schools or child care providers, but it is easier to care for children when there is good communication.
- If parents share information about hepatitis, it should not be shared with staff without written permission of the parents/guardians. Confidentiality should be respected and the plan for sharing information should be very clear to all.

What adaptations may be needed?

Medications

- Do not give any over-the-counter medications such as acetaminophen (eg, Tylenol) or ibuprofen (Motrin is one brand of ibuprofen) to a child with hepatitis without permission from the health care professional.
- Note: Preventive vaccines that protect against hepatitis A and B are available and should be given according to the recommendations of the routine immunization schedule (available online at www.cispimmunize.org, www.aapredbook.org, and www.cdc.gov/vaccines/recs/schedules/default.htm). Immune globulin against hepatitis A may be recommended in outbreak situations.

Dietary considerations

- Because some hepatitis viruses can be spread through saliva, do not share utensils or food from the same plate with a person with viral hepatitis.
- Strict hygiene precautions are required for infectious hepatitis.

➤continued

Hepatitis, continued

- Eating small portions more frequently or eating high-calorie foods may be necessary if weight loss is a problem. Drinking plenty of water is helpful.

Physical environment

- Adaptations will vary depending on the type of hepatitis, whether it is acute or chronic, and whether it is contagious.
- The child may need to limit activities that could lead to abdominal trauma.
- Standard precautions should be followed when blood or blood-containing fluids are handled (for all children, regardless of hepatitis status). For blood and blood-containing substances, these are the same precautions described by the Occupational Safety and Health Administration as universal precautions.
  - ~ Wear disposable gloves or, if using utility gloves, be sure the utility gloves are sanitized after use.
  - ~ Absorb as much of the spill as possible with disposable materials; put the contaminated materials in a plastic bag with a secure tie.
  - ~ Clean contaminated surfaces with detergent and water.
  - ~ Rinse with water.
  - ~ Sanitize the clean surface by wetting the entire surface with a solution of freshly diluted bleach in a 1:10 concentration. Health authorities recommend using a stronger solution of freshly diluted bleach (1:10) to disinfect surfaces that involved blood because if hepatitis B is present, the virus is know to be more resistant to being killed by bleach than many other types of infectious agents.
  - ~ Dispose of all soiled items in plastic bags with secure ties.

What should be considered an emergency?

Call emergency medical services/911 for
- Vomiting blood
- High fever and abdominal pain or swelling
- Confusion or dramatic change of behavior

What types of training or policies are advised?

Standard precautions

What are some resources?

- *Managing Infectious Diseases in Child Care and Schools: A Quick Reference Guide,* 2nd Edition, American Academy of Pediatrics, www.aap.org/bookstore, 888/227-1770
- Centers for Disease Control and Prevention, www.cdc.gov, 800/CDC-INFO (232-4636)

American Academy of Pediatrics

DEDICATED TO THE HEALTH OF ALL CHILDREN™

The information contained in this publication should not be used as a substitute for the medical care and advice of your pediatrician. There may be variations in treatment that your pediatrician may recommend based on individual facts and circumstances.

The American Academy of Pediatrics is an organization of 60,000 primary care pediatricians, pediatric medical subspecialists, and pediatric surgical specialists dedicated to the health, safety, and well-being of infants, children, adolescents, and young adults.

American Academy of Pediatrics
Web site—www.aap.org

Human Immunodeficiency Virus (HIV)

What is human immunodeficiency virus (HIV)?

- Human immunodeficiency virus (HIV) is an infectious disease, but it is included in this book because unlike many infectious diseases, HIV is a lifelong condition for many children.
- HIV is a blood-borne viral infection that attacks the body's immune system. Infection with HIV involves the cells responsible for controlling the body's immune system. Infants and young children usually acquire HIV from their mother when they are born, but with widespread testing and aggressive treatment of infected mothers during their pregnancy, this type of transmission has become much less common.
- HIV is also rarely acquired by contaminated needles or sharp instruments, or through contact of mucous membranes or injured skin with infected substances such as blood or secretions.
- The most common means by which adolescents become HIV-infected is through sexual contact and use of intravenous drugs.

How common is it?

- Approximately 6,100 children and youth who acquired HIV during birth were living in 2006.
- Between 100 and 200 babies are born infected with HIV in the United States each year, despite the availability of HIV testing and treatment.

What are some characteristics of children with HIV?

- Most children with HIV may appear very healthy and be able to participate in all activities. Some children with HIV/AIDS are frequently sick and may require numerous hospitalizations.
- Children with active HIV infection can get
  ~ Diarrhea.
  ~ Swollen lymph nodes.
  ~ Pneumonia and other lung diseases.
  ~ Thrush (a yeast infection on the surfaces of the mouth).
  ~ Babies with HIV may not gain weight well if their disease is not controlled by medication.

Who is the treatment team?

- Infectious disease specialists are frequently involved in the child's health care as well as the primary care provider in the medical home.

- Parents/guardians do not have to share information about the HIV status of their children with schools or child care providers, but it is easier to care for children when there is good communication.
- If parents share the HIV status of their child, the information should not be shared with staff without written permission of the parents/guardians. Confidentiality should be respected and the plan for sharing information should be very clear to all.

What adaptations may be needed?

Medications

- It is very important that children with HIV take their medication regularly. The medications may not taste good but can often be flavored. Ask if the medication can be mixed with pudding or applesauce.
- Exposure to varicella (chickenpox) and measles can be particularly dangerous for children with HIV infection. Make sure that all the children enrolled at the program are up to date on their vaccinations to minimize the risk of these infections. All parents should be notified about an exposure to measles or chickenpox but early, personal notification of parents of children with HIV infection (as for any other immune-deficiency disease), if the identity of these children is known, is recommended.

Physical environment

- Children with HIV can participate in all activities that their health permits. It is important to establish good lines of communication before enrollment to discuss all the relevant health-related issues.
- For all children, regardless of HIV status, standard precautions should be followed when blood or blood-containing fluids are handled. For blood and blood-containing substances, these are the same precautions described by the Occupational Safety and Health Administration as universal precautions.
  ~ Wear disposable gloves or, if using utility gloves, be sure the utility gloves are sanitized after use.
  ~ Absorb as much of the spill as possible with disposable materials; put the contaminated materials in a plastic bag with a secure tie.
  ~ Clean contaminated surfaces with detergent and water.
  ~ Rinse with water.

➤continued

Human Immunodeficiency Virus (HIV), continued

~ Sanitize the clean surface by wetting the entire surface with a spray application of freshly diluted domestic bleach (¼ cup of bleach in 1 gallon of water equals 1 tablespoon to a quart) and leaving this solution in contact with the surface for at least 2 minutes. Some health authorities recommend using a stronger solution of freshly diluted bleach (1:10) to disinfect surfaces that involved blood because if hepatitis B virus is present, it is more difficult to kill with bleach than other organisms that might be found in blood. HIV is easily deactivated by bleach.

~ Dispose of all soiled items in plastic bags with secure ties.

What should be considered an emergency?

- There are no special emergencies faced by children with HIV that vary from other children.
- Notify parents immediately for exposure to chickenpox or measles.
- Biting of another child or vice versa.

What types of training or policies are advised?

- Standard precautions
- Biting

What are some resources?

- *Managing Infectious Diseases in Child Care and Schools: A Quick Reference Guide,* 2nd Edition, American Academy of Pediatrics, www.aap.org/bookstore, 888/227-1770
- Centers for Disease Control and Prevention, www.cdc.gov, 800/CDC-INFO (232-4636)
- *Caring for Our Children: National Health and Safety Performance Standards: Guidelines for Out-of-Home Child Care Programs,* 2nd Edition, standards 3.026, 3.027, 6.033, 6.034, 8.053, and 8.057

American Academy
of Pediatrics

DEDICATED TO THE HEALTH OF ALL CHILDREN™

Hydrocephalus and Shunts

What is hydrocephalus?

Hydrocephalus is the abnormal accumulation of spinal fluid, called *cerebrospinal fluid* (CSF), within the brain. Hydrocephalus can be caused by a structural defect in the brain or spine that blocks CSF and causes it to accumulate. Sometimes a brain injury, especially one that causes bleeding, can interfere with the flow of CSF and cause it to build up and increase pressure. Sometimes, the brain can shrink because of brain damage and the CSF fills in the extra space. That condition does not cause pressure on the brain and does not require special treatment.

What are shunts?

One treatment of hydrocephalus is the placement of a *shunt,* which is a flexible tube, to carry the extra CSF from the ventricle of the brain to another area of the body. A successful shunt system allows an infant's head size to become normal and relieves pressure on the brain. A ventriculoperitoneal shunt carries CSF into the peritoneal or abdominal cavity.

What are some characteristics of children with hydrocephalus or shunts?

- A shunt can be seen as a tube tunneled under the skin from the head to the chest or abdomen. Often, there is a flexible plastic pump located on the head.
- Shunt tubes may require replacement as a child grows. Successful shunts usually are maintained for life, but there can be complications such as
  - ~ Mechanical failure, infections, and obstructions.
  - ~ Tubes that need to be lengthened or replaced.
  - ~ Shunt systems requiring monitoring and regular medical follow-up. When complications happen, a shunt usually requires some type of revision.
- Many children with hydrocephalus have normal intelligence, but some may experience developmental delays or have an intellectual disability.
- Hydrocephalus may be an isolated problem or it may be related to another condition such as spina bifida.

Who is the treatment team?

- The treatment team consists of the child's primary care provider in the medical home, pediatric neurosurgeon, and physical, speech, and occupational therapists.

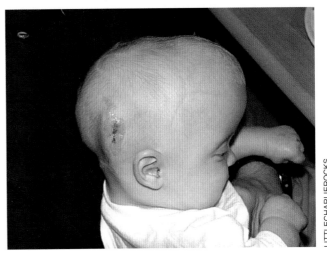
Child with a shunt to drain excess fluid

LITTLECHARLIEROCKS

- Children who are younger than 3 years may receive therapy through *early intervention* services. Therapists working with early intervention may interact with caregivers/teachers after the child has shunt surgery.
- Older children may get services through *special education and related services.*

What adaptations may be needed?

Physical environment

There are generally no limitations to activity in a child with a shunt in place, although some surgeons ask the child to refrain from contact sports in which there might be a physical blow to the pump or tubing at the head.

What should be considered an emergency?

- Call parents for any early signs of shunt malfunction or infection.
  - ~ Fever
  - ~ Vomiting
  - ~ Irritability or lethargy
  - ~ Redness or swelling along the shunt tract
  - ~ Vision problems
  - ~ Loss of coordination or balance
  - ~ Headache
  - ~ Dizziness
  - ~ Sensitivity to light

➤continued

Hydrocephalus and Shunts, continued

- Call emergency medical services/911 and arrange for the child to be transported to a neurosurgical center for
  - ~ Seizures
  - ~ Extreme lethargy
  - ~ Loss of consciousness
  - ~ Behavior change
  - ~ Severe headache with vomiting

What types of training or policies are advised?

- Caring for children with shunts
- Recognizing signs and symptoms of shunt failure

What are some resources?

Spina Bifida Association, 800/621-3141, www.sbaa.org

American Academy
of Pediatrics

DEDICATED TO THE HEALTH OF ALL CHILDREN™

The information contained in this publication should not be used as a substitute for the medical care and advice of your pediatrician. There may be variations in treatment that your pediatrician may recommend based on individual facts and circumstances.

The American Academy of Pediatrics is an organization of 60,000 primary care pediatricians, pediatric medical subspecialists, and pediatric surgical specialists dedicated to the health, safety, and well-being of infants, children, adolescents, and young adults.

American Academy of Pediatrics
Web site—www.aap.org

Idiopathic Thrombocytopenic Purpura

What is idiopathic thrombocytopenic purpura?

- Idiopathic thrombocytopenic purpura (ITP) is a bleeding disorder caused by having too few platelets in the blood. Platelets are small cells in the blood that help to form blood clots, which stop bleeding.
- No one knows exactly why ITP occurs, but the immune system begins to attack its own platelets. It may be triggered by the aftereffects of a viral infection. It often goes away on its own.
- It must be distinguished from more serious conditions. Unlike many conditions discussed in this book, ITP is more likely to develop in a child while in child care or school rather than be a preexisting condition.
- Expected course
  - ~ Within 3 months, 75% of patients have recovered.
  - ~ By a year, 90% have a normal platelet count.
  - ~ A few children go on to have more chronic cases.
  - ~ The risk of bleeding may be related to the platelet count.

What are some characteristics of children with idiopathic thrombocytopenic purpura?

- Idiopathic thrombocytopenic purpura can start with purple bruising (purpura) or a characteristic type of pinpoint bleeding called petechiae.
- Nosebleeds or oral bleeding are also common ways for ITP to present.
- The child may also have blood in the urine or the stools.
- Because it presents as unexplained bruising, there may be a concern about child abuse before the condition is diagnosed. However, ITP is not caused by physical abuse.
- Children generally appear healthy despite their bruises and are often remarkably resistant to bruising despite very low platelet counts

Who is the treatment team?

The treatment team may consist of the primary care provider and a hematologist.

What adaptations may be needed?

Medications

- Many times, no medications need to be given.
- Sometimes ITP is treated with steroids or immune therapy.
  - ~ Immune therapy is usually given in a health care setting.
  - ~ Steroids can usually be given at home but the side effects of steroids, which include mood changes, increased appetite, nausea, weight gain, and behavior changes, might be seen while the child is in child care or school.
- Rarely, the spleen needs to be removed.
- All children with clotting disorders should avoid nonsteroidal anti-inflammatory drugs such as ibuprofen (with brand names such as Advil or Motrin), naproxen (eg, Aleve), and aspirin.
- Acetaminophen, with brand names such as Tylenol, is usually fine to use, but patients with bleeding disorders should discuss any medications to be taken with their physicians and health care professionals, even over-the-counter medicines.

Dietary considerations

There is no special diet for ITP, but hard foods that could cut the mouth should be avoided.

Physical environment

- Scheduling a visit with parents/guardians before the child returns to the program to review specifics of their child's condition can be helpful.
- Avoid head trauma and limit climbing. A child with ITP may need to stay home until the condition is under control. Precautions include ensuring straps in high chairs are fastened and sharp corners are padded.

What should be considered an emergency?

- Call emergency medical services/911 for
  - ~ Uncontrolled bleeding, including a nosebleed that doesn't stop after 15 minutes
  - ~ Headache
  - ~ Inability to move a body part
  - ~ Change in behavior
  - ~ Difficulty speaking
  - ~ Loss of consciousness

➤continued

Idiopathic Thrombocytopenic Purpura, continued

- Call parents/guardians for
  - ~ Increased bruising
  - ~ Minor bleeding that is controlled with first aid

What types of training or policies are advised?

- First aid to stop bleeding
- Standard precautions
- Background about ITP

What are some resources?

National Heart, Lung and Blood Institute, www.nhlbi.nih.gov

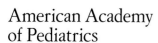

American Academy
of Pediatrics

DEDICATED TO THE HEALTH OF ALL CHILDREN™

Kidney/Urinary Problems

What are kidney/urinary problems?

- Urinary problems may include the kidneys, bladder, or ureters.
  - ~ The kidneys are 2 fist-sized organs in the back of the abdomen that are responsible for filtering the blood and removing waste products.
  - ~ Ureters are tubes that carry the urine from the kidneys to the bladder.
  - ~ The bladder sits right above the pubic bone and collects the urine.
- This Quick Reference Sheet will provide information on nephrotic syndrome, nephritis (glomerulonephritis), and recurrent urinary tract infections (UTIs).
  - ~ Nephrotic syndrome and nephritis (glomerulonephritis) are kidney problems.
  - ~ Recurrent UTIs affect the bladder, but the ureters or kidneys may also be involved.
- Occasionally, children will have renal (kidney) failure and may need to get some form of dialysis.
  - ~ Dialysis is a procedure that removes waste products from the blood.
  - ~ Dialysis can occur through the blood or abdomen.

Who is the treatment team?

- In general, kidney and urinary problems are handled in the child's medical home.
- If subspecialty consultation is required, it is usually provided by a pediatric nephrologist or pediatric urologist.
- Surgery of the urinary system is usually performed by a pediatric urologist.

What are some related Quick Reference Sheets?

- Altered Immunity: An Overview (page 59)
- "Hypertension (High Blood Pressure)" section of Heart Conditions, Functional (page 103)

What are some resources?

- National Kidney and Urologic Diseases Information Clearinghouse, nkudic@info.niddk.nih.gov
- National Kidney Foundation, www.kidney.org

Nephrotic Syndrome

What is nephrotic syndrome?

- Nephrotic syndrome is caused when protein leaks through the membranes in the kidney.
- Without the protein, fluid escapes out of the blood vessels and into the body tissue, which causes swelling, especially of the legs, abdomen, and face.
- There can be dramatic weight gain from the water and the child may urinate less.
- The cause is unknown.
- There are several types of nephrotic syndrome, but the most common in childhood is minimal change disease. The outlook for children with minimal change disease is quite good, and the vast majority of children recover from minimal change nephrotic syndrome without any permanent kidney damage.

What are some characteristics of children with nephrotic syndrome?

Nephrotic syndrome can occur at any age but is most common between the ages of 18 months and 8 years. Boys are affected more often than girls. A child may come to the child care or school with the diagnosis or may develop it while enrolled.

What adaptations may be needed?

Medications
- Treatment often starts with steroids.
  - ~ If the nephrotic syndrome is controlled with steroids, they should be slowly discontinued.
  - ~ Steroids may need to be given again if there is a relapse. Sometimes the disease comes back when the steroids are tapered and different medications may need to be considered.
  - ~ Side effects from steroids may include mood swings, increased appetite, and weight gain (which can be hard to sort out from the fluid weight).
  - ~ Over a longer period, steroids can suppress the immune system and make the child more vulnerable to infection.
- Diuretics (fluid pills) are also used to decrease the amount of fluid in the body. Because of the recurrent nature of this condition and the need to repeatedly alter steroid dosages or add additional medications, these children are often referred to a pediatric nephrologist.

➤*continued*

- While the disease is active, the immune system is weakened for 2 reasons.
  - ~ First, the body is not making proteins and is also losing proteins, which help to fight infection
  - ~ Second, steroids can also suppress the immune system.
  - ~ It is important for the child to avoid exposure to chickenpox and measles at those times.
- Because nephrotic syndrome can come and go, at times it is necessary to check the urine for protein. This is done with a urine dipstick that changes colors if dipped in urine that contains protein. The Care Plan should specify if this is necessary.
- All over-the-counter medications should be approved by the child's health care professional and specified in the Care Plan.
- Note on vaccinations: Some changes in the vaccine schedule may need to be made because of nephrotic syndrome or the medications used to treat it. The child should have a medical note explaining any necessary changes.
  - ~ It is critical that children with kidney disease be immunized as fully as possible to protect them against any vaccine-preventable diseases.
  - ~ All children should be vaccinated, especially against influenza, but it is particularly important for those with kidney disease.

Dietary considerations

- To prevent swelling and discomfort, a low-salt diet is a vital part of the care of these children.
- Foods containing caffeine such as chocolate, tea, and coffee should be avoided if high blood pressure is part of the condition.

What should be considered an emergency?

Check with the child's Care Plan. Emergencies include
- *Fever.* Because the child's immune system might not be functioning properly, fever can be a serious symptom.
- *Increased swelling.* This might signal worsening of the disease.
  - ~ *Blood clots.* Isolated swelling, color change, or pain in a limb may be a symptom of a blood clot.
  - ~ Abdominal pain or swelling of the abdomen.

What types of training or policies are advised?

- Recognizing symptoms of worsening disease or complication
- Urine testing if that is a part of the child's Care Plan
- Dietary changes

Nephritis (Glomerulonephritis)

What is nephritis (glomerulonephritis)?

- This kidney condition is similar to nephrotic syndrome except the kidneys lose blood and protein in the urine.
- Nephritis can be acute or chronic.
  - ~ The acute form frequently occurs after a strep throat infection. While acute glomerulonephritis usually resolves, there can be complications during the acute phase, and these children should be under the close supervision of their health care professional.
  - ~ The chronic form has more causes and is more problematic.

What are some characteristics of children with nephritis (glomerulonephritis)?

- Children may have swelling and red or brown color of the urine because of blood loss.
- High blood pressure is more common with this form of kidney disease.

How common is it?

Nephritis (glomerulonephritis) is less common than nephrotic syndrome.

What adaptations may be needed?

Considerations are similar to those listed in nephrotic syndrome. Because there are more different types of nephritis, it is important to have a detailed Care Plan that specifies what the particular child needs.

Recurrent Urinary Tract Infections

What are recurrent urinary tract infections?

- Children can get a single UTI, but those who get them repeatedly may have a problem called vesicoureteral reflux.
- With this problem, the urine travels backwards from the bladder toward the kidney. This can cause bacteria to be washed up the urinary tract toward the kidney, where it can do damage. If the urine backs up too far, it may cause swelling of the kidneys or *hydronephrosis.*
- Some children are prescribed a low-dose antibiotic to try to prevent UTIs. Often, children outgrow this problem and then stop taking antibiotics.
- Children are usually born with urinary reflux, but it may take time to diagnose the condition.

➤*continued*

Kidney/Urinary Problems, continued

- Other conditions can cause blockage of the flow of urine but are less likely to cause problems that need to be addressed in child care and school. These include ureteral-pelvic junction obstruction, ureterocele, and posterior urethral valves, which are often surgically corrected in boys shortly after birth. These conditions will not be addressed in this Quick Reference Sheet.

What are some characteristics of children with recurrent urinary tract infections?

Symptoms of a UTI include
- Fever
- Painful urination
- Blood in the urine
- Sensation that they have to urinate even when the bladder isn't full
- Change in the appearance or smell of the urine

What adaptations may be needed?

Medications

Antibiotic prophylaxis (daily low-dose antibiotics) may be recommended. This can usually be administered by parents at home.

Dietary considerations

Hydration is very important for children with UTIs. Children should drink 8 to 10 glasses of water or other fluid per day.

Physical environment

- Change diapers frequently in infants and toddlers.
- Encourage children to use the bathroom every 3 to 4 hours to help wash out the bacteria. Children often get busy with their play and don't remember to go.

What should be considered an emergency?

High fever in the absence of other signs or symptoms may be caused by a kidney infection. Call parents/guardians immediately.

What types of training or policies are advised?

Recognizing symptoms of a UTI

American Academy
of Pediatrics

DEDICATED TO THE HEALTH OF ALL CHILDREN™

Premature Newborns (Preemies): An Overview

What is a premature newborn (preemie)?

- Premature newborns (preemies) are babies who are born early. A premature newborn is one who is born before 37 weeks of pregnancy; a preemie can be very early (after only 6 months of pregnancy) or older (after 8 months), but both may have problems that result in the need for specialized care.
- Many newborns who are born prematurely will need neonatal intensive care after birth, and some continue to face challenges or health issues throughout childhood.

How common is premature birth?

One in 8 babies (12.7%) was born prematurely (less than 37 weeks' gestation) in 2005. Of live births, 2% were born very preterm (less than 32 weeks).

What are some characteristics of premature newborns?

Some of the most common long-term problems faced by preemies are

- Lungs
  - ~ The lungs of premature newborns are often not ready to function and can suffer damage during necessary treatment. This form of lung disease is called bronchopulmonary dysplasia (BPD). Many very premature babies with BPD will be discharged from the hospital with supplemental oxygen, often to be used for 6 to 12 months.
  - ~ Parents and care providers need to learn how to use oxygen tanks and associated monitors as they provide these newborns with usual life experiences.
  - ~ Long-term treatment of BPD overlaps with asthma treatment. (See Asthma on page 65 for more details.)
- Apnea
  - ~ When a baby stops breathing, it is called apnea. Premature babies can have apnea because the part of the brain responsible for breathing is immature.
  - ~ In most cases, apnea goes away when newborns reach the age when they would have been born (40 weeks after conception). Rarely does this problem continue after hospital discharge, but in selected cases, babies may be sent home on an apnea monitor, which sounds an alarm warning for changes in breathing or heart rate.
  - ~ Sometimes apnea can be related to gastroesophageal reflux, which requires specific treatment. (See Gastroesophageal Reflux Disease [GERD] on page 91 for more details.)

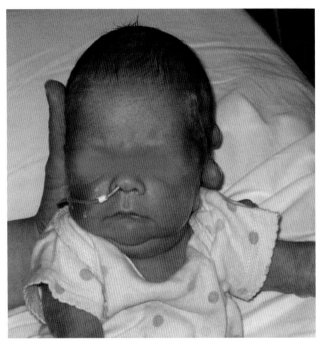

Premature baby

- Central nervous system
  - ~ Some babies may have brain injuries associated with premature birth, including bleeding into the brain, which can lead to hydrocephalus (water on the brain), cerebral palsy, or other developmental disabilities.
  - ~ All premature newborns need close monitoring for developmental problems during infancy and some may need specialized therapies to improve their functional ability. Please see Cerebral Palsy on page 79 and Hydrocephalus and Shunts on page 111 for more information.
- Vision
  - ~ There can be an overgrowth of blood vessels in the back of the eye in premature newborns that can pull on the delicate lining of the eye called the retina. The retina is the part of the eye responsible for vision.
  - ~ Sometimes this condition resolves on its own as the baby grows; sometimes it causes permanent vision loss.
  - ~ Babies may require laser surgery to stabilize the condition. Even those preemies who do not require surgery have an increased need for glasses as they get older.
  - ~ Premature newborns should have regularly scheduled eye examinations throughout infancy and childhood. (See Visual Impairments on page 139 for more details.)

➤continued

- Hearing
  - ~ Premature newborns face multiple risk factors for hearing loss. Most babies have their hearing tested before they leave the neonatal intensive care unit (NICU), but they may need periodic testing as they get older as well. (See Hearing Loss and Deafness on page 95 for more details.)
- Gastrointestinal
  - ~ Some babies have an intestinal infection in the NICU that can damage the bowel, and sections of bowel may need to be surgically removed. This can leave a baby with short gut syndrome, which makes it hard for the newborn to digest food properly.
  - ~ Babies with short gut may need small, frequent feedings and a special diet.
- Blood
  - ~ Some premature newborns become anemic (low red blood cell count). They may require blood transfusions while in the NICU or may need iron and extra vitamins.
- Nutrition
  - ~ Preemies frequently need special formula or fortified breast milk early on to grow properly.
  - ~ Some babies continue to have growth and feeding challenges that may require occupational, speech, or feeding therapies, and in some cases, use of feeding devices.
- Infection
  - ~ Preemies may be vulnerable to infections in the first year of life. The most serious are usually viral infections such as flu or respiratory syncytial virus (RSV) that attack the lungs.
- Development
  - ~ The development of premature babies can vary.
  - ~ Some preemies catch up quickly and do things like walk and talk at the same time as their peers who were born at term after a full 9 months. Others may lag behind their peers until 2 or 3 years of age.
  - ~ Some preemies have permanent neurologic damage and developmental delays, which are usually apparent early in infancy.
  - ~ Other preemies, without clearly defined neurologic injuries, show more subtle educational and behavioral problems as they get older. Early childhood experiences may lessen the risk of these problems.
  - ~ Preemies may be small for their age and have long, narrow heads from the pressure on the soft skull bones.
  - ~ Some preemies are poor feeders and grow slowly in weight and height.

Who is the treatment team?

- Preemies will often be followed by a special neonatal follow-up team at the hospital where they were in the NICU. Neonatal follow-up teams might include neonatologists, developmental specialists, and neonatal nurse practitioners.
- Speech, occupational, physical, and respiratory therapists might also be involved in the baby's care.
- Social workers are available to help parents cope with family and social issues.
- These teams may monitor preemies for developmental delays or apnea, or might give special medications like those listed under "Medications."
- Preemies might need to see subspecialists such as pediatric ophthalmologists (eye doctors), pulmonologists (lung doctors), neurologists (brain doctors), or gastroenterologists (stomach and intestine doctors).
- Audiologists (hearing specialists) may be needed to monitor hearing over time.

What adaptations may be needed?

Medications

- Premature newborns should receive immunizations on the same schedule as their term peers.
- In addition, they may receive special injections (palivizumab/Synagis) during winter months for their first year to strengthen their immune system's ability to fight off RSV.
- There are no other routine medications given to premature infants, but those with BPD may receive medications for wheezing, diuretics (water pills), and supplemental oxygen.

Dietary considerations

- Give preemies extra time to eat and digest their food if necessary.
- Some preemies may be on special infant formulas or breast milk fortifiers.

Physical environment

- Find out from parents what challenges their child had from being born prematurely and what challenges still exist.
- Check out the Quick Reference Sheets in this book related to the specific problem that the child still faces such as apnea, GERD, cerebral palsy, or visual or hearing impairments.
- Exposure to colds and respiratory illnesses can be a problem for premature babies with lung disease. Preemies without lung disease will likely do better when faced with respiratory infections. With premature newborns with lung

➤continued

disease, the family may want to consider using small group care to limit the child's exposure to respiratory illnesses in the first year of life. When this is not possible, measures such as cohorting a small group of infants with a primary caregiver in a separate space could be considered. Evidence for the effectiveness of these measures is lacking. Avoid secondary smoke exposure for all infants, but particularly for preemies with vulnerable lungs.

- Premature newborns are at increased risk for sudden infant death syndrome (SIDS). Be sure to place babies to sleep on their backs. A preemie may be even more susceptible to SIDS when placed asleep on his tummy than a term baby.
- Remember to adjust developmental expectations to account for the baby's prematurity (eg, a baby born 2 months early should be acting like a 4-month-old when she is 6 months old).
- Let parents/guardians know if the program staff has any concerns about a baby's hearing or vision, especially if the baby was born prematurely.

What should be considered an emergency?

Premature babies often have a complex medical history after a long newborn hospitalization. Assessment during an emergency department visit may be difficult if that background information is not readily available. The program should have a copy of pertinent medical history in the event the child must be taken to the hospital for immediate evaluation.

What types of training or policies are advised?

- Pediatric first aid training that includes CPR (management of a blocked airway and rescue breathing) with instructional demonstration and return demonstration by participants on a manikin. *Pediatric First Aid for Caregivers and Teachers* is a course designed to teach these skills.
- Specific training related to care, especially apnea monitor training.

What are some resources?

- March of Dimes, www.marchofdimes.com
- Linden DW, Paroli ET, Doron MW. *Preemies: The Essential Guide for Parents of Premature Babies.* New York, NY: Pocket Books; 2000
- Emory University School of Medicine Developmental Progress Clinic On-line Resource Center, www.pediatrics.emory.edu/neonatology/dpc

Seizures, Febrile

What are febrile seizures?

Febrile seizures are described as generalized (whole brain and body involved), tonic-clonic (shaking) movements of a child's body in response to a high fever. These seizures represent abnormal brain electrical activity triggered by fever.

How common are they?

Febrile seizures are very common, occurring in up to 2% to 4% of all children during the early childhood years. These occur normally in children between 6 months and 6 years of age, with the majority of children experiencing their first febrile seizure at a median age of 15 to 21 months.

What are some characteristics of children with febrile seizures?

- Typical febrile seizures cause generalized shaking of the body lasting 1 to 2 minutes, with a rapid return to consciousness.
  - ~ These seizures tend to occur with a rapid rise in body temperature and usually happen only once during any given illness.
  - ~ Often febrile seizures happen at the start of an illness, sometimes before the fever is even apparent.
- Atypical febrile seizures are different from typical seizures in the following ways:
  - ~ Seizure is prolonged and may last longer than 15 minutes.
  - ~ Seizure is focal, or partial, and involves just part of the body.
  - ~ A child experiences more than one seizure during the same febrile illness.
  - ~ A child younger than 6 months or older than 6 years.
  - ~ A child with preexistent neurologic or developmental problems.
  - ~ A strong family history for epilepsy.
- Most children who have febrile seizures are developmentally and intellectually normal. About 25% of these children will have a family history of febrile seizures.

Who is the treatment team?

- Specialists, such as neurologists or developmental pediatricians, are rarely involved in the management of these children, which is very different than children who have seizures without fever.

- Brain studies such as magnetic resonance imaging or computed tomography scanning and electroencephalogram are generally not indicated and if done, are typically normal in children with simple febrile seizures.

What are some elements of a Care Plan for febrile seizures?

How to keep a child safe during a seizure—the emergency Care Plan
- Call 911.
- Keep calm. You cannot stop a seizure once it has started. Let the seizure run its course. Do not try to revive the child.
- Ease the child to the floor and loosen his clothing.
- Try to remove any hard, sharp, or hot objects that might injure the child. You may place a cushion or soft item under his head.
- Turn the child to his side, so that saliva can flow out of his mouth.
- Protect the breathing passages by tilting the head back a bit and adjusting the jaw forward in the sniffing position.
- Do not put anything in the child's mouth. He may bite his tongue, but that will not stop him from breathing.
- Try to time the seizure and note what parts of the body are involved. This information may be helpful to physicians caring for the child afterward.
- After the seizure, let him rest if he is sleeping.
- Contact his parents/guardians.
- If the child wakes after the seizure, he may be groggy or irritable, and just needs comfort measures.

What adaptations may be needed?

Medications

- The Care Plan should include having fever-reducing medications such as acetaminophen (eg, Tylenol) or ibuprofen (eg, Motrin, Advil) on hand in case the child develops a fever in the center or school. This medication can be supplied by the parent, but instructions for using the medication should be written out for the program staff by a health care professional.
- Unfortunately, simple medicines to reduce the fever (antipyretics) have not been shown to prevent febrile seizures.
- When a child has a fever, the fever is not an illness. The source of the fever must be identified.

➤continued

Seizures, Febrile, continued

- Some children will have rectal suppositories (eg, rectal diazepam gel) prescribed to be given if the child develops a febrile seizure. These medications can help stop or shorten a seizure, but in some cases, they can slow breathing. If a seizure medication is to be used by program staff, the plan for using the medication should be discussed with the parents and prescribing physician to make sure the plan, including how to monitor and manage any medication side effects, are completely understood.
- Some centers or schools prefer to hold seizure medication and allow emergency medical technicians to administer it if necessary.
- Call parents if the child develops a fever or any other illness symptom.
- Seizures often scare people who do not know about them but usually will not harm the child who has one. A febrile seizure doesn't cause brain damage.

What should be considered an emergency?

Call emergency medical services/911 if
- The seizure lasts longer than 10 minutes.
- The child has a series of short seizures.
- The child is injured during the seizure.
- This is the child's first seizure.

What types of training or policies are advised?

- Medication administration
- CPR
- Emergency preparation

What are some resources?

- National Institute of Neurological Disorders and Stroke, 800/352-9424, www.ninds.nih.gov
- Epilepsy Foundation, 800/332-1000, www.epilepsyfoundation.org

American Academy
of Pediatrics

DEDICATED TO THE HEALTH OF ALL CHILDREN™

Seizures, Non-febrile (Epilepsy)

What are non-febrile seizures (epilepsy)?

- Seizures are sudden abnormal events or episodes that happen because of a problem with the way brain cells communicate through electrical signals.
- During a seizure, some brain cells send abnormal and exaggerated electrical signals that stop other cells from working properly.
- A seizure causes the patient to experience temporary disturbances in awareness or consciousness, movement, sensation, and behavior.

How common are they?

Seizures represent the most common neurologic disorder in children. About 1% of all children have a type of non-febrile seizure disorder, or epilepsy.

What are some characteristics of children with non-febrile seizures?

- Different types of seizures represent different parts of brain involvement.
  - ~ *Generalized* (formerly known also as *grand mal*) seizures occur when the whole brain and whole body are involved. A child may stiffen and shake all over in a rhythmic or biphasic *tonic* (stiff) *clonic* (jerking) fashion. Children may fall to the ground and hurt themselves during a seizure. Sometimes they lose control of their bladder or bowels. Most seizures last no more than 3 or 4 minutes. Children do not respond to you during these seizures and may be very confused and sleepy afterward for hours.
  - ~ *Absence* (known as *petit mal*) seizures look like staring spells. These children may stop and stare for a few seconds in the middle of whatever they are doing. The child who is having an absence seizure will not be able to respond to you while it is happening and will have no memory of the episode afterward. There may be lip smacking or rhythmic eye blinking while the child is not responsive.
  - ~ *Partial* seizures can be simple or complex because only a part of the brain is involved.
    - ❖ In a *simple partial* seizure, a child may do many things such as shake one part of his body or see, hear, or smell something that is not there. The child is not confused during these episodes, although he may be frightened.
    - ❖ During a *complex partial* seizure, a child may be confused or have a distortion of consciousness. During these episodes, children may behave in a strange way or may have strange words or actions such as hand rubbing, lip smacking, or swallowing. They are confused and sleepy after the seizure is over.
- Many children with seizures have normal intelligence; some have developmental delays.

Who is the treatment team?

- A pediatric neurologist often directs the medical management of children with seizures.
- Children with developmental delays may receive speech, occupational, or physical therapy.
- Children younger than 3 years may receive these therapies through *early intervention* services. These therapists may suggest activities or exercises that could be helpful in the child's Care Plan.

What are some elements of a Care Plan for non-febrile seizures?

- Call 911.
- Activate emergency medical services (EMS).
- Emergency plans—how to keep a child safe during a seizure
  - ~ Keep calm. You cannot stop a seizure once it has started. Let the seizure run its course and say comforting, soothing things to the child.
  - ~ Ease the child to the floor and loosen her clothing.
  - ~ Try to remove any hard, sharp, or hot objects that might injure the child. You may place a cushion or soft item under her head.
  - ~ Turn the child to her side, so that saliva can flow out of her mouth.
  - ~ Do not put anything in the child's mouth. She may bite her tongue, but that will not stop her from breathing,
  - ~ After the seizure, let her rest if she is sleeping. Contact her parents/guardians.
  - ~ If the child wakes after the seizure, she may be groggy or irritable and just needs comfort measures.

►*continued*

Seizures, Non-febrile (Epilepsy), continued

What adaptations may be needed?

Medications

- Many children with non-febrile seizures take medication for their seizure disorder, and medication administration may be part of their Care Plan. These medications are often called *anticonvulsants;* there are many different types.
  - ~ Talk to parents/guardians about the child's particular anticonvulsant therapy and the side effects that might be associated with the medication, especially those affecting learning and attention.
  - ~ Most anticonvulsants suppress seizures, but the medication may not be able to completely eliminate all seizure activity.
- Some children will have rectal suppositories (eg, rectal diazepam gel) prescribed to be given if the child develops a febrile seizure. These medications can help stop or shorten a seizure, but in some cases, they can slow breathing. If a seizure medication is to be used by program staff, the plan for using the medication should be discussed by the program staff with the parents and prescribing physician. This helps to ensure that the plan, including how to monitor and manage any medication side effects, is completely understood.
- Some centers or schools prefer to hold seizure medication and allow emergency medical technicians to administer it if necessary.
- Many seizure medications have interactions with other types of medications, so make sure to check before giving a child on anticonvulsants any over-the-counter medications.

Dietary considerations

Some children with seizures may be on a special diet known as the ketogenic diet. Parents/guardians or a dietitian can give you details on the diet if necessary.

Physical environment

- Communicate with the child's parents/guardians and doctor about the individual type of seizure, medications, and emergency plan. Update this on a regular basis, preferably after the child has his neurology appointments.
- Children may be more prone to seizures when they are ill. Unusual irritability, lethargy, or fevers are cues to alert the child's parents/guardians.
- Children may have triggers to seizures, such as flashing lights, lack of sleep, or eating poorly. Discuss seizure triggers with the child's parents/guardians.
- Seizures often scare people who do not know about them, but usually they will not harm the child who has one.

What should be considered an emergency?

- Call parents/guardians for
  - ~ Change in the child's activity or behavior
  - ~ Increased staring or single muscle jerks
  - ~ Fever
- Call EMS/911 for seizures unless staff is trained and comfortable with handling seizure. In that case, the child's Care Plan should specify when to call 911 for a seizure.

What types of training or policies are advised?

- CPR
- First aid
- Medication administration
- Policy on seizures and emergencies

What are some resources?

Epilepsy Foundation, 800/332-1000, www.epilepsyfoundation.org

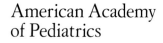

American Academy of Pediatrics

DEDICATED TO THE HEALTH OF ALL CHILDREN™

Sickle Cell Disease

What is sickle cell disease?

- Sickle cell is a condition in which red blood cells change shape. Instead of being round and smooth, they form a "c" shape like a crescent moon (see Figure at right). They can get stuck in blood vessels and block blood flow, which can cause pain or swelling and keep the body from fighting infection.
- The abnormally shaped red blood cells do not live as long as regular cells, so children with sickle cell disease have a low blood count and must make new red blood cells more quickly.
- Children are born with this condition and have it for life. Some children are more severely affected; some have a milder form.

How common is it?

- There are about 72,000 people in the United States with sickle cell disease. It is most common in people of African or Mediterranean descent.
- People with sickle cell *trait* do not have the disease and are generally healthy. Children with sickle cell trait usually have no special requirements. About 2 million Americans have sickle cell trait.

What are some characteristics of children with sickle cell disease?

- Children with sickle cell disease may have a yellow tint to their eyes because of a by-product of the breakdown of red blood cells. They may be small or slender for their age.
- Children with sickle cell disease may have increased absences because of complications and may need to be hospitalized for treatment. Some complications include
  ~ Pain
    ❖ Pain can happen in any part of the body but often occurs in the hands, feet, or joints.
    ❖ Chest pain can be especially serious. Signs of acute chest syndrome include cough, difficulty breathing, and fever.
  ~ Fever
    ❖ Children with sickle cell disease can have a hard time fighting infection. The abnormal cells can interfere with the body's ability to clear out and destroy bacteria.
    ❖ Fevers must be evaluated urgently by the child's health care professional. Treatment includes laboratory blood studies and antibiotic administration to avoid complications.
    ❖ Pneumonia can be very serious in children with sickle cell disease.
  ~ Splenic sequestration
    ❖ Splenic sequestration is an emergency.
    ❖ The spleen is an organ in the upper left section of our abdomen next to the stomach. The spleen acts to strain the blood and remove damaged cells and infection. Sickled cells can clog up the spleen and keep it from working properly. Sometimes sickled cells get especially clogged in the spleen and cause the blood to back up. The spleen can get very big if this happens and can sometimes break open, which is a life-threatening emergency.
  ~ Aplastic crisis
    ❖ Abnormal blood cells have a shorter lifespan, so the body needs to make new blood cells very quickly. If something such as a viral infection prevents the body from keeping up with making new blood cells, cell count can drop and the child can get a dangerously low blood count very quickly. If this happens, the child can appear very pale and tired.
  ~ Strokes
    ❖ If sickled cells block the blood flow to the brain, a stroke can occur.
    ❖ Signs include headache, weakness of a body part, seizure, or speech problems.
    ❖ Strokes require emergency evaluation and treatment.
  ~ Skin ulcers
    ❖ These need to be treated promptly if they develop.
  ~ Priapism
    ❖ Boys with sickle cell disease may get painful penile erections related to poor blood flow that require emergency treatment.
- Some children with more severe disease require regular blood transfusions.
- There are other blood diseases that may share some characteristics of sickle cell disease. These are called hemoglobinopathies, in which red blood cell proteins are abnormal.

Who is the treatment team?

- Children with sickle cell disease may have their primary medical care with the primary care provider in their medical home or with a specialty clinic. Check with parents/guardians about who the first point of contact should be.
- Hematologists are the specialists who care for children with blood diseases.

➤*continued*

Sickle Cell Disease, continued

What adaptations may be needed?

Medications

- Children with sickle cell may take penicillin from 2 months until 5 years of age to help prevent infection. Erythromycin may be substituted in children who are allergic to penicillin. Pain crisis is treated with medications like acetaminophen (eg, Tylenol), codeine, and ibuprofen (eg, Motrin, Advil). Extra amounts of folic acid may be required because of the extra red blood cells that are needed.
- Note on vaccinations: Children with sickle cell disease may need special vaccines such as pneumococcal or early meningococcal as well as routine immunizations. All children should receive annual flu vaccinations, but this is especially important for children with sickle cell disease.

Dietary considerations

Children with sickle cell disease should have at least 8 cups of water or fluid per day.

Physical environment

- Hydration helps to prevent sickling, so allowing the child to have a water bottle is a good idea.
- Children with sickle cell disease may need increased bathroom breaks.
- Most children with sickle cell disease have normal activity, but allow them to rest if they tire easily with anemia.
- Avoid extreme temperatures, hot and cold.

Transportation Considerations

Special consideration should be given to transport to and from child care or school because vehicles can be very warm or cold, either of which can increase sickling of red cells.

What should be considered an emergency?

- Call parents/guardians immediately for
  - ~ Fever
  - ~ Pain that does not improve with medication and rest
  - ~ Cough or mild chest pain
  - ~ Abdominal pain or swelling
  - ~ Paleness or increased tiredness
  - ~ Painful erection
- Call emergency medical services/911 if
  - ~ Difficulty breathing.
  - ~ Seizure or loss of consciousness.
  - ~ Headache or dizziness.
  - ~ Change in vision.
  - ~ Numbness or inability to move a body part.
  - ~ Severe pain.
  - ~ The spleen gets enlarged (sequestration).
  - ~ Prolonged erection.

What types of training or policies are advised?

- Recognizing impending crisis and signs and symptoms of complications
- Responding to emergencies
- Medication administration

What are some resources?

- The Sickle Cell Information Center, www.scinfo.org/teacher.htm
- National Heart, Lung and Blood Institute, www.nhlbi.nih.gov
- Regional sickle cell centers (contact local resources or children's hospitals for more information)

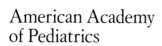

American Academy
of Pediatrics

DEDICATED TO THE HEALTH OF ALL CHILDREN™

The information contained in this publication should not be used as a substitute for the medical care and advice of your pediatrician. There may be variations in treatment that your pediatrician may recommend based on individual facts and circumstances.

The American Academy of Pediatrics is an organization of 60,000 primary care pediatricians, pediatric medical subspecialists, and pediatric surgical specialists dedicated to the health, safety, and well-being of infants, children, adolescents, and young adults.

American Academy of Pediatrics
Web site—www.aap.org

Special Diets and Inborn Errors of Metabolism

What are special diets and inborn errors of metabolism?

- Inborn errors of metabolism are rare genetic disorders in which the body lacks the protein (enzyme) to turn certain foods into energy normally. Foods that are not broken down to produce energy can build up in a child's system and cause illness, low blood sugar, intellectual disability, and death.
- The most common inborn error of metabolism is phenylketonuria.

How common are they?

Some of the more common inborn errors of metabolism include
- Phenylketonuria, 1 in 19,000 live births
- Medium-chain acyl-CoA dehydrogenase deficiency, 1 in 23,000 live births
- Homocystinuria, 1 in 39,000 live births
- Galactosemia, 1 in 55,000 live births
- Biotinidase deficiency, 1 in 95,000 live births

What are some characteristics of children with special diets or inborn errors of metabolism?

- Most of these children look normal at birth. However, within the first few days of life they may look jaundiced, and have trouble feeding and persistent vomiting.
- They may appear irritable or lethargic.
- Some of these children have a peculiar odor that may range from smelling like maple syrup (maple syrup urine disease) to sweaty socks (isovaleric acidemia).
- Many of these conditions are tested in the newborn screening program and can be diagnosed shortly after birth.
- Once diagnosed, the baby must be placed on a very strict diet. This diet prevents the accumulation of any substance that might build up in the child's body and cause harm.
- Often special formulas are used beyond infancy into childhood. If the child keeps the offending food out of his diet, he may grow and develop normally.

Who is the treatment team?

- Children with inborn errors of metabolism require close supervision by a primary care provider in the medical home and registered dietitian and geneticist. The Care Plan essentially involves dietary measures and should be directed by these professionals with guidance from the child's parents/guardians.
- The Care Plan should have emergency measures for when these children begin to appear ill.

What adaptations may be needed?

Dietary considerations

- Meet with parents/guardians prior to the child's arrival to school or child care to discuss dietary measures in detail.
- Meet periodically with parents/guardians, especially at transition times (eg, infancy to toddlerhood, preschool to school age) to discuss new dietary plans.
- Ask parents/guardians to suggest or provide acceptable treats for their child for class parties and birthdays.
- As children notice differences in what this child can eat, use this as a teachable moment to discuss nutrition and foods that are good for growing bodies.

What should be considered an emergency?

- Inform parents/guardians immediately if the child
  ~ Has repetitive episodes of vomiting.
  ~ Acts unusually irritable or lethargic.
- Parents/guardians, together with the treatment team, should provide the indications for calling emergency medical services/911.
- Children with some inborn errors of metabolism may have much more devastating consequences than others when they are ill, and an emergency plan is necessary.

What types of training or policies are advised?

Dietary

What are some resources?

National Organization for Rare Disorders, 800/999-NORD (999-6673), www.rarediseases.org

American Academy of Pediatrics

DEDICATED TO THE HEALTH OF ALL CHILDREN™

Spina Bifida

What is spina bifida?

Spina bifida means cleft spine, which is an incomplete closure in the spinal column. The 4 types of spina bifida are

- Spina bifida occulta
  - ~ There is an opening in one or more of the vertebrae (bones) of the spinal column without damage to the spinal cord.
- Occult spinal dysraphism (OSD)
  - ~ The child has minor abnormality of the skin overlying the lower spine, such as a hairy patch, pigmented area, or small opening (sinus).
  - ~ The spinal cord below this abnormality is at high risk for injury as the child grows; evaluation of the spinal cord (eg, with a magnetic resonance imaging scan) should be performed.
- Meningocele
  - ~ The meninges, the protective covering around the spinal cord, have pushed out through the opening in the vertebrae in a sac called the meningocele. However, the spinal cord remains intact.
  - ~ This form can be repaired with little or no damage to the nerve pathways.
- Myelomeningocele
  - ~ This is the most severe form of spina bifida, in which a portion of the spinal cord itself protrudes through the back.
  - ~ In some cases, sacs are covered with skin; in others, tissue and nerves are exposed.
  - ~ Generally, people use the terms spina bifida and myelomeningocele interchangeably.

How common is it?

- The most severe forms occur in approximately 1 out of every 1,000 births.
- Of these newborns, the majority (94%) have myelomeningocele, and the rest (6%) have meningocele and OSD.

What are some characteristics of children with spina bifida?

- *Muscle weakness.* Children with myelomeningocele usually have muscle weakness or paralysis below the area of the spine where the incomplete closure (or cleft) occurs.
- *Sensation disturbances.* Children may need wheelchairs or may be able to use crutches or walkers. Children usually do not feel sensation in the limbs or body parts below the cleft.
- *Bowel and bladder problems.* Children with spina bifida often do not develop normal bowel and bladder control. Many children with myelomeningocele need training to learn to manage their bowel and bladder functions. Some require *catheterization,* the insertion of a tube to permit passage of urine.
- *Latex allergy.* Many children with spina bifida are allergic to latex or are at risk for becoming allergic.
- *Hydrocephalus.* In addition, this condition may cause an accumulation of fluid in the brain, or hydrocephalus. (See Hydrocephalus and Shunts on page 111 for more details.)
  - ~ It is estimated that 70% to 90% of children born with myelomeningocele have hydrocephalus.
  - ~ The higher the abnormality is on the spine, the greater the risk for hydrocephalus.
  - ~ Hydrocephalus is controlled by a surgical procedure called shunting, which relieves the fluid buildup in the brain.
  - ~ Before shunting, most children born with a myelomeningocele died shortly after birth. Now that surgery to drain spinal fluid and protect children against hydrocephalus can be performed in the first 48 hours of life, children with myelomeningocele are much more likely to live.
  - ~ Quite often, however, they must have a series of operations, including shunt revisions, throughout their childhood.
- *Vision problem.* Children with spina bifida may have problems with their eyes or vision.

Who is the treatment team?

- Many pediatric specialists are involved in the care of children with spina bifida. Pediatric neurosurgeons and orthopedic surgeons, neurologists, gastroenterologists, and urologists often work together in a *multispecialty center* to address and coordinate the medical needs of these children.
- Many children with spina bifida benefit from *physical therapy, occupational therapy,* or *speech therapy* to learn adaptive skills and how to function with their peers.
- Children who are younger than 3 years may receive these therapies through *early intervention* services. Early intervention is a system of services to support infants and toddlers with disabilities and their families.
- For children 3 years and older, *special education and related services* are available through the public school to provide the therapies necessary for school achievement.

➤continued

Spina Bifida, continued

What are some elements of a Care Plan for spina bifida?

- Care Plans for children with spina bifida often include *intermittent catheterization,* a procedure in which a tube is placed in the bladder and urine is drained.
- The Care Plan may also incorporate physical or occupational therapy exercises into a daily routine.
- These plans may include the use of splints, braces, communication devices, or adapted toys to help children be more active, participate more, and have fun while they are working their bodies.
- Exposure to latex (eg, rubber-containing toys, bandages) should always be limited.
- A written plan called the Individualized Family Service Plan will be provided for children in early intervention.
- An Individualized Education Program will describe an older child's unique needs and the services available to address them.
- These children should have at least one visit with a qualified eye specialist.

What adaptations may be needed?

Physical environment

- Many children learn self-intermittent catheterization at an early age, sometimes as young as 5 years. A private area in which this can be done will be helpful.
- A successful bladder management program can be incorporated into the school day or child care program.
- Architectural factors need to be considered when caring for a child with spina bifida. Ramps, ground-floor entrances, and wheelchair-accessible areas may be needed.
- Children with hydrocephalus as part of their spina bifida often have learning disabilities or attention deficits.
- Children with spina bifida have varying physical capabilities and limitations. Work with the child's family and therapists on goals to improve the child's mobility without increasing the child's or family's frustration with the child's limitations.

What should be considered an emergency?

- If the child has a seizure, follow emergency guidelines for seizures (see page 123).
- Notify parents/guardians of
  - ~ Fever
  - ~ Severe headache, lethargy, irritability, or new crossing of eyes
  - ~ Numbness or tingling in limbs
  - ~ Any loss of function, eg, weakness in legs
  - ~ Inability to obtain urine with catheterization
- Children with spina bifida may need extra time, supervision, or transport in case of an emergency such as a fire.
- Any critical adaptive equipment would also need to be brought in the event of an evacuation.

What types of training or policies are advised?

- Catheterization
- Care Plan specifics
- Safe transfer or transportation

What are some resources?

- Spina Bifida Association, 800/621-3141, www.sbaa.org
- National Dissemination Center for Children with Disabilities, 800/695-0285 (voice/TTY), www.nichcy.org

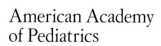

American Academy
of Pediatrics

DEDICATED TO THE HEALTH OF ALL CHILDREN™

Spleen Problems

What are spleen problems?

- The spleen is an organ is the upper left section of the abdomen near the stomach.
- The spleen is responsible for producing and filtering out red blood cells. It is also a part of the immune system, which protects against infection.
- It is an important organ but is not critical to survival.

How common are they?

Because the spleen can be affected differently by different diseases, it is difficult to say how many children have spleen problems.

What are some characteristics of children with spleen problems?

- Other conditions mentioned in this book may affect the spleen, such as sickle cell and other blood diseases, or cancer.
- The spleen can also be enlarged temporarily in infectious mononucleosis or HIV.
- Sometimes the spleen is injured during trauma and must be removed surgically.
- Some children are born with abnormal spleens.
- The spleen can be a problem if it is enlarged, does not work properly, or is missing.

What adaptations may be needed?

Medications

- The spleen filters out bacteria. If it is not working well, the body can get an overwhelming infection very quickly. Certain vaccines, such as pneumococcal and meningococcal, help to prevent infections. Influenza vaccine can also be helpful.
- Some children take penicillin to prevent overwhelming bacterial infections.
- Fever can be a more serious symptom and should be evaluated by a health care professional capable of doing blood studies for and administering antibiotics to a child with an absent or a nonfunctioning spleen.

Physical environment

Enlarged spleens may be at risk for rupturing (breaking open), which is a life-threatening emergency. Therefore, it is important to avoid hitting the abdomen in rough play or sports activities. Sometimes the cause of an enlarged spleen is temporary, such as infectious mononucleosis, and sometimes it is chronic, such as some blood diseases.

What should be considered an emergency?

- Call emergency medical services/911 for
  ~ Serious pain in the left upper abdomen
  ~ A child who appears pale or weak
  ~ Fever if the parent cannot take the child for immediate evaluation
  ~ Serious trauma to the abdomen in a child known to have an enlarged spleen
  ~ Enlarging spleen (belly swelling)
- Call parents/guardians for
  ~ Fever, if the Care Plan specifies that the parent will take the child for evaluation and the parent is able to do so
  ~ Decreased energy
  ~ Minor abdominal pain or discomfort
  ~ Minor abdominal trauma

What types of training or policies are advised?

Recognizing signs and symptoms of possible emergency

What are some resources?

Emergency information form (see "Emergency Information Form for Children With Special Needs" in Chapter 11 on page 159)

American Academy of Pediatrics

DEDICATED TO THE HEALTH OF ALL CHILDREN™

Tracheostomy

What is a tracheostomy?

- A tracheostomy is a surgical opening made in the neck into the trachea (windpipe) that allows a child to breathe without using the nose or mouth.
- A tracheostomy tube is inserted into the opening to allow breathing and removal of secretions. There are several different types.
  - *Single cannula.* This type is generally seen in infants and small children. These may or may not have a *cuff* to hold them in place.
  - *Double cannula.* This type has an inner lining and an outer, removable piece. It is usually held to the child by laces or a Velcro-fastened neck band called *trach* (pronounced "trake") *ties.*
  - *Cuffed.* A cuffed tube has a soft balloon around the distal (far) end that can be inflated to seal the space around the tube against the trachea to allow for mechanical ventilation (use of a respirator) in patients with respiratory failure. The cuff is inflated with air, foam, or sterile water.
  - *Fenestrated.* A fenestrated tube has an opening in the tube that permits speech when the external opening of the tracheostomy tube is blocked with a finger or special speaking valve. The opening in the part of the tube that is inside the trachea allows air to pass into the upper airway across the vocal folds to make speech sounds. These tubes are usually not used in younger children

How common is it?

- A tracheostomy tube is placed in children for many reasons, including birth defects, complications of prematurity, feeding problems, and brain disorders.
- More children are receiving tracheostomies because lifesaving medical treatments are now available that allow children to survive serious medical conditions.

Who is the treatment team?

- Primary care provider in the medical home.
- A pediatric pulmonologist and surgeon may be involved in the child's care.
- A respiratory therapist may also be involved if the child is on a ventilator.
- Some children have home nurses who may accompany them to school or child care.

What are some elements of a Care Plan for a child with a tracheostomy?

The Care Plan should address
- Suctioning of the tracheostomy
  - A clean disposable suction tube placed in the child's tracheostomy tube is hooked up to a suction machine to remove any of the child's secretions that have built up and might block the child's breathing.
  - This may be done up to every 4 hours and is usually done by the child's nurse.
- Eating
  - Children with tracheostomies generally can eat by mouth. A few children also have eating or swallowing problems that will be addressed in the Care Plan.
  - Most children do require suctioning prior to eating and may require suctioning after eating if any food slips down into the airway.
  - Plenty of fluids are recommended to keep secretions thin and moist.
- Speech
  - There are many ways in which a child with a tracheostomy can speak.
    - ❖ Certain types of tracheostomy tubes.
    - ❖ Special speaking valves that allow air into the tube, but block air from going out except through the upper airway (eg, Passy-Muir valve).
    - ❖ Plugging the trachea with a finger temporarily will encourage speech.
- Children younger than 3 years may receive speech therapy through *early intervention* services. Early intervention is a system of services to support infants and toddlers with disabilities and their families.
- For children 3 years and older, *special education and related services* are available through the public school to provide the therapies necessary for school achievement.

What adaptations may be needed?

Physical environment

- When holding a child with a tracheostomy, be sure the chin is up and the tube opening is unobstructed.
- Prevent foreign objects from entering the tracheostomy tube, such as water, sand, dust, and small toy pieces.
- Avoid sandboxes and beaches.
- Avoid chalk dust.

➤*continued*

Tracheostomy, continued

- Watch play with other children so that toys, fingers, and food are not put into the tracheostomy tube and that other children don't pull on the tube.
- Avoid clothing that blocks the tracheostomy tube, such as crewnecks, turtlenecks, and shirts that button in the back.
- No plastic bibs.
- No necklaces.
- No fuzzy or fur clothing or stuffed toys.
- Do not allow anyone to smoke near the child.
- No latex balloons—these are dangerous for all children. Latex over any airway will block breathing.
- Avoid exposure to people with colds or other contagious illnesses to the extent possible.

What should be considered an emergency?

- Call emergency medical services/911 for
  - ~ Difficulty breathing, especially if accompanied by noisy breathing (grunting or whistling from the tube) or cyanosis (pale, blue color of lips and skin).
  - ~ Increased respiratory rate or effort.
  - ~ Sweaty, clammy skin.
  - ~ Retractions—extra work of breathing that involves pulling in of the skin between the ribs, below the breastbone, above the collarbones, or in the hollow of the neck.
  - ~ Tracheostomy tube comes out and cannot be replaced.
  - ~ Extreme restlessness or change in level of consciousness (eg, sudden lethargy, not responding).
- Notify parents/guardians for
  - ~ Fever and increased secretions
  - ~ Redness, rash, or foul odor at the tracheostomy site

What types of training or policies are advised?

There must be a trained person with the child at all times who is able to identify an emergency and
- Suction and replace a tracheostomy tube that is blocked with secretions.
- Ventilate the child using an oxygen bag.
- Perform CPR.
- For children who are transported, there should be a trained person (preferably a registered nurse or licensed practical nurse) with the child at school and on the bus to and from the program.

What are some resources?

- Cynthia Bisscll, RN, Aaron's Tracheostomy Page, www.tracheostomy.com
- American Thoracic Society, 212/315-8600, www.thoracic.org

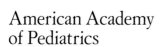

American Academy
of Pediatrics

DEDICATED TO THE HEALTH OF ALL CHILDREN™

Turner Syndrome

What is Turner syndrome?

Turner syndrome is a genetic condition that only affects girls and women. It occurs when 1 of the 2 X chromosomes normally found in females is missing or incomplete.

How common is it?

- Turner syndrome is very common, occurring in about 1 out of 2,500 live births.
- Approximately 800 infants are diagnosed each year, and 60,000 girls and women in the United States are affected.

What are some characteristics of children with Turner syndrome?

- The most common characteristics of Turner syndrome include
  - ~ Short stature
  - ~ Arms that turn out slightly at the elbows
  - ~ Webbed neck
  - ~ Low hairline in the back of the head
  - ~ Puffy hands and feet, known as lymphedema
- Possible complications of Turner syndrome include
  - ~ Congenital heart disease, especially coarctation (narrowing) of the aorta.
  - ~ Gastroesophageal reflux (increased spitting), and difficulty growing and gaining weight.
  - ~ Thyroid problems.
  - ~ Kidney problems.
  - ~ Frequent ear infections.
  - ~ Normal intelligence, but often learning disabilities (eg, visual-spatial weakness; problems with copying designs, right/left directions, math).
  - ~ Younger children may have increased anxiety.
  - ~ Orthopedic problems including dislocated hips and scoliosis (curvature of the spine).

Who is the treatment team?

- The treatment team for children with Turner syndrome includes the primary care provider in the medical home and pediatric specialists in genetics, endocrinology, orthopedics, and sometimes cardiology.

- Physical therapy may be necessary for children with orthopedic problems.
- Special education targeted at visual-spatial weaknesses and counseling for anxiety may be needed.

What adaptations may be needed?

Medications

There are no special medications needed for Turner syndrome, but the Care Plan may include medications or special exercises for these children if they have other conditions (eg, heart conditions). See Heart Conditions, Functional, on page 101 for more details.

Physical environment

- Avoid placing infants in backpack carriers, umbrella strollers, walkers, or jumpers because these can increase reflux.
- Many children will appear younger than their age because of their short stature. Be sure to take their age into account as you interact with them.
- Infants may need *reflux precautions,* which are measures to keep them from spitting up or vomiting their food. These precautions can include things such as keeping the child upright after feedings, frequent burping, and sleeping with the head of the bed angled up.
- Many children are at risk for teasing because of their physical appearance. Work to foster self-confidence with the child, as well as understanding among her classmates.

What should be considered an emergency?

No special emergency planning is needed for girls with Turner syndrome unless the child has other related conditions.

What are some resources?

- Turner Syndrome Society of the United States, 800/365-9944, www.turnersyndrome.org
- Frías JL, Davenport ML, American Academy of Pediatrics Committee on Genetics, Section on Endocrinology. Health supervision for children with Turner syndrome. *Pediatrics.* 2003;111:692–702

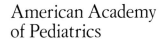

American Academy of Pediatrics

DEDICATED TO THE HEALTH OF ALL CHILDREN™

Visual Impairments

What are visual impairments?

- Visual impairments are present when a child cannot see well enough to interact with others and participate in daily child care or school activities (at her developmental level).
- Partially sighted, low vision, and legally blind are terms used to describe the different levels of visual impairment related to a child's needs in child care or another educational setting.
  - ~ A child who is *partially sighted* has a visual problem that requires some special accommodations in child care and school. These children may need glasses at an early age.
  - ~ A child with *low vision* has a severe visual impairment. They can see shapes and people around them, but most everything will be fuzzy, even with glasses. They require a fair amount of accommodation and assistance, and may need to be taught to read using braille. An infant or a young child would need specialized or expert care in a child care setting.
  - ~ A child who is *legally blind* has very limited vision or a severely constricted visual field, and might not see anything at all. Students who are totally blind learn via braille or other nonvisual means, usually in special settings or with one-on-one assistance. Students with a severely constricted visual field may be able to read but still need special accommodations in child care and school.

How common are they?

- The rate at which visual impairments occur in children aged 0 to 18 years is 12.2 per 1,000.
- Severe visual impairments (legally or totally blind) occur in children aged 0 to 18 years at the rate of 0.06 per 1,000.

What are some characteristics of children with visual impairments?

- Children with visual impairments usually have many eye and other conditions. Often, it is those conditions that led to visual impairments.
  - ~ These problems include retinopathy of prematurity, albinism, cataracts, glaucoma, tumors, congenital infections and disorders, and diabetes.
  - ~ The effect of visual problems on a child's development depends on the severity of the problem, level of visual impairment, age at which the condition appears, and services offered to the child.
  - ~ Children who have visual impairment as one of multiple disabilities may have significant developmental problems.
- If a child with a visual impairment is diagnosed in infancy and treatment begins early, he will most likely do well and learn to use his other senses to adapt to his environments.
- Because a child who has severe visual impairments cannot see his parents/guardians, caregivers/teachers, or peers, he may not imitate social behavior or understand nonverbal cues. This can make it harder to become self-sufficient and independent. Because children's sense of self-worth develops during the years they may be in child care and school, it is extremely important that others who interact with a child with a visual impairment support that child and help him to feel good about what he can do, celebrate his accomplishments, and value him as a whole person.

Who is the treatment team?

- The treatment team for a child with a visual impairment can include the primary care provider in the medical home, a pediatric ophthalmologist (an eye doctor who mostly works with children), developmental and behavioral pediatricians, vision specialists, and child development experts or early childhood educators.
- A young child with visual impairment may not explore her environment in the same way a child who can see would. Special accommodations and *early intervention* are important and necessary.
  - ~ Early intervention is a state-funded system of services to support infants and toddlers with disabilities and their families.
  - ~ Therapists and other professionals that are part of the early intervention system can work with caregivers/teachers to incorporate exercises and equipment into the day-to-day lives of these young children.
  - ~ For children 3 years and older, *special education and related services* are available through the public school to provide therapies necessary for school achievement.
- Often the local Commission for the Blind works with the child and family to assist with specific home, child care, and school adaptations.

➤*continued*

Visual Impairments, continued

What adaptations may be needed?

Dietary considerations

- There are no special dietary considerations, but it is helpful to establish consistent place settings and expectations around eating.
- Help children anticipate that there may be spills and teach them how to handle this themselves, as well as to ask for help when they need it.

Physical environment

- Provide plenty of light.
- Keep the furniture and supplies in the same place in the classroom. Sharp objects such as scissors and art supplies should be kept in an enclosed container. Also maintain a very consistent routine. This will help all children, especially those with a visual impairment, to feel more comfortable because they will know what to expect and where things are.
- Provide a safe environment by keeping drawers and cabinet doors closed as well as keeping traffic patterns free of toys, throw rugs, electrical cords, or other objects that might be hard to see or move around. Orient the child to locations of steps and stairs. Teach the child to use handrails.
- Establish barrier-free routes in the area where the child spends time and within the facility, such as from the classroom to the bathroom. Use contrasting colors, such as a green plate on a white tablecloth. (It is difficult to see a white plate on a white cloth.)
- Use sounds and auditory cues to help children understand what is going on and what will happen next; eg, say what you are doing, use songs or music for transitions from one activity to another. Model for the other children in the classroom how they can do this in a sensitive way too.
- Directly supervising children by sight and sound is best, especially in child care programs. However, if you have to leave an older child with a visual impairment alone, have the child stand near a wall, railing, chair, or something else to hold on to until you return. Leaving the child alone in an open space may create anxiety and confusion. Again, explain what you are doing as you do it.

- Allow children to experience leadership opportunities within the classroom, as this will foster self-confidence and independence.
- A Care Plan for a child with a visual impairment may include specific information for caregivers/teachers or the child to help emphasize listening skills, communication choices, ways to handle new situations or settings, and moving from one place to another.
- Technology such as computers and low-vision optical aids and videos may enable children with visual impairments to participate more fully in classroom activities.
- Use books in braille as well as those with large print or on a tape.

What should be considered an emergency?

- There are not many medical emergencies that children with visual impairments would typically experience, but extra time and supervision will be necessary in the event of an evacuation for a programmatic emergency such as a fire. This should be taken into consideration in emergency planning, and all children should know what to expect and how they can help the child with visual impairments and each other.
- Children with visual impairments are at greater risk for falls and non-intentional injuries (eg, banging into furniture, tripping). Prevention of these events is a crucial component of the Care Plan.

What are some resources?

- Blind Childrens Center, 323/664-2153, www.blindchildrenscenter.org
- National Association for Parents of Children with Visual Impairments, 800/562-6265, www.napvi.org
- Commission for the Blind (in various states; contact local health resources for more information)

American Academy
of Pediatrics

DEDICATED TO THE HEALTH OF ALL CHILDREN™

CHAPTER 11

Sample Documents and Forms

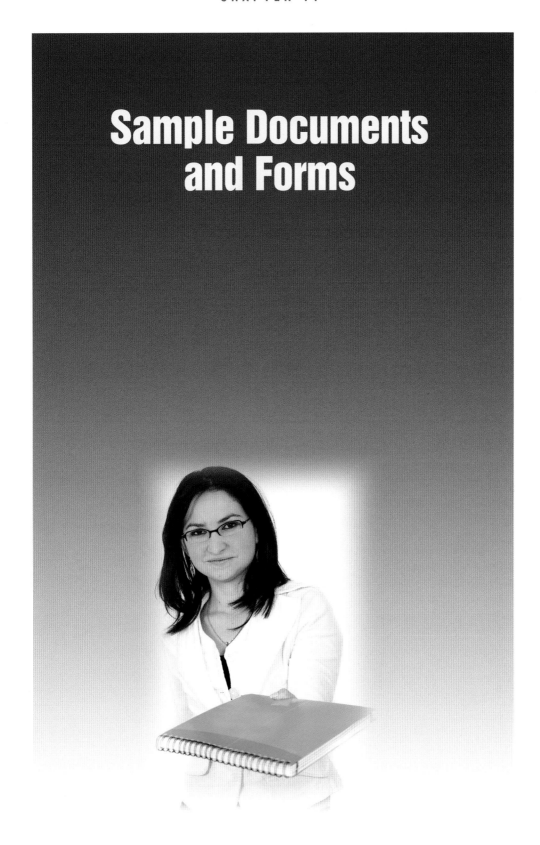

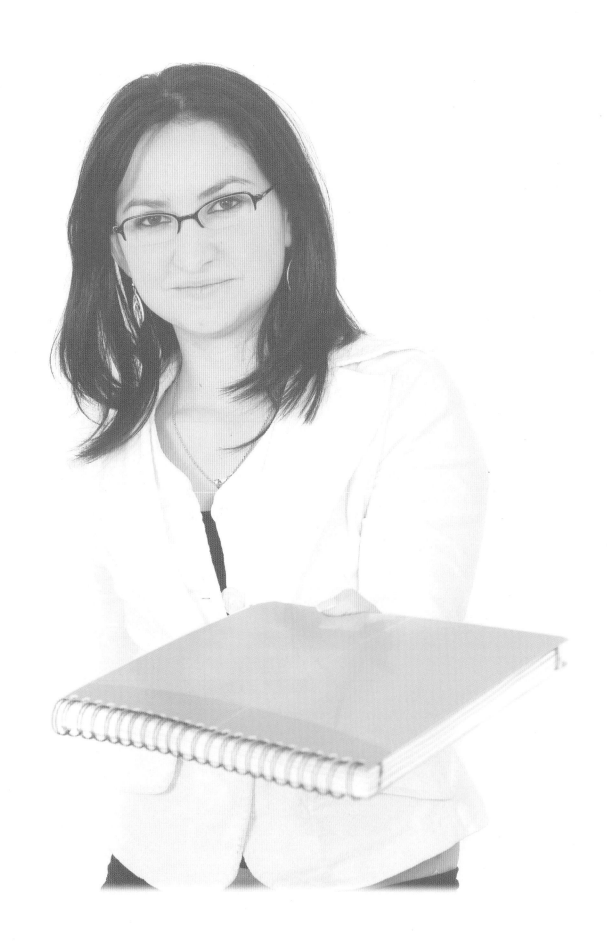

Sample Documents and Forms

See earlier chapters for how these documents and forms can be used, as well as strategies for using them.

Copy or adapt these sample documents and forms to facilitate communication among parents, caregivers/teachers, and pediatric health professionals. Some of the samples are state-specific and included for example purposes. No permission is necessary to make single copies for noncommercial, educational purposes.

Medication Administration Packet

Authorization to Give Medicine
PAGE 1—TO BE COMPLETED BY PARENT

CHILD'S INFORMATION

Name of Facility/School

_____/_____/_____
Today's Date

Name of Child (First and Last)

_____/_____/_____
Date of Birth

Name of Medicine _____

Reason medicine is needed during school hours _____

Dose _____   Route _____

Time to give medicine _____

Additional instructions _____

Date to start medicine _____/_____/_____   Stop date _____/_____/_____

Known side effects of medicine _____

Plan of management of side effects _____

Child allergies _____

PRESCRIBER'S INFORMATION

Prescribing Health Professional's Name

Phone Number

PERMISSION TO GIVE MEDICINE

I hereby give permission for the facility/school to administer medicine as prescribed above. **I also give permission for the caregiver/teacher to contact the prescribing health professional about the administration of this medicine. I have administered at least one dose of medicine to my child without adverse effects.**

Parent or Guardian Name (Print)

Parent or Guardian Signature

Address

Home Phone Number   Work Phone Number   Cell Phone Number

Adapted with permission from the NC Division of Child Development to the Department of Maternal and Child Health at the University of North Carolina at Chapel Hill, Connecticut Department of Public Health, and Healthy Child Care Pennsylvania.

Receiving Medication
PAGE 2—TO BE COMPLETED BY CAREGIVER/TEACHER

Name of child _____

Name of medicine _____

Date medicine was received _____/_____/_____

Safety Check

- ☐   1. Child-resistant container.

- ☐   2. Original prescription or manufacturer's label with the name and strength of the medicine.

- ☐   3. Name of child on container is correct (first and last names).

- ☐   4. Current date on prescription/expiration label covers period when medicine is to be given.

- ☐   5. Name and phone number of licensed health care professional who ordered medicine is on container or on file.

- ☐   6. Copy of Child Health Record is on file.

- ☐   7. Instructions are clear for dose, route, and time to give medicine.

- ☐   8. Instructions are clear for storage (eg, temperature) and medicine has been safely stored.

- ☐   9. Child has had a previous trial dose.

Y ☐   N ☐   10. Is this a controlled substance? If yes, special storage and log may be needed.

_____
Caregiver/Teacher Name (Print)

_____
Caregiver/Teacher Signature

Medication Log
PAGE 3—TO BE COMPLETED BY CAREGIVER/TEACHER

Name of child _____ Weight of child_____

	Monday	Tuesday	Wednesday	Thursday	Friday
Medicine					
Date	/ /	/ /	/ /	/ /	/ /
Actual time given	AM _____ PM _____	AM _____ PM _____	AM _____ PM _____	AM _____ PM _____	AM _____ PM _____
Dosage/amount					
Route					
Staff signature					

	Monday	Tuesday	Wednesday	Thursday	Friday
Medicine					
Date	/ /	/ /	/ /	/ /	/ /
Actual time given	AM _____ PM _____	AM _____ PM _____	AM _____ PM _____	AM _____ PM _____	AM _____ PM _____
Dosage/amount					
Route					
Staff signature					

Describe error/problem in detail in a Medical Incident Form. Observations can be noted here.

Date/time	Error/problem/reaction to medication	Action taken	Name of parent/guardian notified and time/date	Caregiver/teacher signature

	Date	Parent/guardian signature	Caregiver/teacher signature
RETURNED to parent/guardian	/ /		
	Date	Caregiver/teacher signature	Witness signature
DISPOSED of medicine	/ /		

Medication Incident Report

Date of report _____ School/center _____

Name of person completing this report _____

Signature of person completing this report _____

Child's name _____

Date of birth _____ Classroom/grade _____

Date incident occurred _____ Time noted _____

Person administering medication _____

Prescribing health care provider _____

Name of medication _____

Dose _____ Scheduled time _____

Describe the incident and how it occurred (wrong child, medication, dose, time, or route?)

_____

_____

_____

Action taken/intervention _____

Parent/guardian notified?   Yes _____   No _____   Date _____   Time _____

Name of the parent/guardian that was notified _____

Follow-up and outcome _____

Administrator's signature _____

Adapted with permission from Healthy Child Care Colorado.

Preparing to Give Medication

This is a checklist to use at your child care facility/school to make sure that your program is ready to give medication. There is also a Receiving Medication checklist (page 146) with more detail to use whenever a parent drops off medication.

1. Paperwork

☐ Parent authorization to give medications is signed.

☐ Health care professional authorization or instructions are on file.

☐ Child Health Record is on file.

2. Medication checked when received

☐ Properly labeled.

☐ Proper container.

☐ Stored correctly.

☐ Instructions are clear.

☐ Disposal plan is developed.

3. Administering medication

☐ Area is clean and quiet.

☐ Staff is trained.

☐ Hands are washed.

☐ The 5 rights are followed—right child, medication, dose, time, and route.

☐ Child is observed for side effects.

4. Documentation

☐ Medication log is completed fully and in ink.

Adapted with permission from the NC Division of Child Development to the Department of Maternal and Child Health at the University of North Carolina at Chapel Hill.

Information Exchange on Children With Health Concerns Form

Dear Health Care Provider:

We are sending you this Information Exchange Form along with a Consent for Release of Information Form (see back) because we have a concern about the following signs and symptoms that we and/or the parents have noted in this child, who is in our care. We appreciate any information you can share with us on this child in order to help us care for him/her more appropriately, and to assist us to work more effectively with the child and family. Thank you!

To be filled out by Child Care Provider:

Facility Name: _____ Telephone: _____

Address: _____

We would like you to evaluate and give us information on the following signs and symptoms: _____

_____

_____

_____

Questions we have regarding these signs and symptoms are: _____

_____

_____

_____

Date____/___/___   Child Care Provider Signature: _____

                        Child Care Provider Printed Name: _____

To be filled out by Health Care Provider:

Health Care Provider's Name: _____ Telephone: _____

Address: _____

Diagnosis for this child: _____

Recommended Treatment: _____

_____

_____

_____

Major side effects of any medication prescribed that we should be aware of: _____

_____

Should the child be temporarily excluded from care, and if so, for how long? _____

_____

What should we be aware of in caring for this child at our facility (special diet, treatment, education for parents to reinforce your instructions, signs and symptoms to watch for, etc.)?

_____

_____

_____

Please attach additional pages for any other information, if necessary.

Date____/___/___   Health Care Provider Signature: _____

                        Health Care Provider Printed Name: _____

California Childcare Health Program   www.ucsfchildcarehealth.org   rev. 04/05

Consent for Release of Information Form

I, _____, give my permission for

(parent/guardian)

_____ to exchange health information with

(sending professional/agency)

_____.

(receiving professional/agency)

This includes access to information from my child's medical record that is pertinent to my child's health and

safety. This consent is voluntary and I understand that I can withdraw my consent for my child at any time.

This information will be used to plan and coordinate the care of:

Name of Child: _____   Date of Birth: _____

Parent/Guardian Name: _____

(print full name)

Parent/Guardian Signature: _____

**Parents or Guardians signing this document have a legal right
to receive a copy of this authorization.**

Note: In accordance with the Health Insurance Portability and Accountability Act (HIPAA) and applicable local laws,
all personal and health information is private and must be protected.

Adapted from: Pennsylvania Chapter of the American Academy of Pediatrics (1993). Model Child Care Health Policies.
Bryn Mawr: PA: Authors.

California Childcare Health Program   www.ucsfchildcarehealth.org   rev. 10/03

Parent/Health Professional Release Form

Authorization for Release of Information

I, _____ , give permission for
(parent/guardian)

_____
(health professional/facility)

to release to _____ the following information:
(facility/school)

_____ .
(screenings, tests, diagnoses, treatments, recommendations)

The information will be used solely to plan and coordinate the care of my child, kept confidential, and only shared with _____

_____ .
(staff title/name)

Name of Child _____ _____

Address _____

City _____ State _____ Zip _____

Date of Birth _____

_____
Parent/Guardian Signature

_____
Witness Signature

_____
Staff Member to Contact for Additional Information

Sample Consent Form to Obtain Health Insurance Portability and Accountability Act (HIPAA) Privacy-Protected Information From a Child's Physician or Primary Health Care Provider

I authorize _____ to use and/or disclose protected health information about
(physician/provider)

_____ in communications with the following individual or entity:
(child)

_____
(specific contact or contacts at child care program/school)

_____
(address)

_____
(address)

_____
(city, state, zip)

_____   _____   _____
(telephone)   (fax)   (e-mail)

The protected health information covered by this authorization includes the following:
• Health status of the child listed, including immunizations given and screening test results
• Health problems/conditions pertinent to the child's enrollment in a child care program/school
• Recommendations for care that would assist caregivers/teachers to meet the needs of the child or could affect the care of other children/adults with whom the child has contact

Check one:
☐ This authorization will expire on _____.
(date)

☐ This authorization will expire when I provide written notice to all individuals listed.

I understand that information regarding my child will only be shared with the individuals listed on this form. If a need to disclose information to others is identified, another form will need to be completed/filed. I have the right to revoke this authorization for future communications any time that I provide written/dated notice to all individuals listed. I understand that I cannot revoke this authorization when disclosure has already occurred as described in this form.

_____
(Print Name of Parent or Legal Guardian)

_____
(Signature of Parent or Legal Guardian)

_____
(Street or PO Box)

_____
(City, State, Zip)

_____
(Telephone)

_____
(Date Parent or Legal Guardian Signed This Form)

Emergency Information Form for Children With Special Needs

■■■ American College of
■■■ Emergency Physicians®

American Academy
of Pediatrics

Date form completed	Revised	Initials
By Whom	Revised	Initials

Name:	Birth date:	Nickname:

Home Address:	Home/Work Phone:
Parent/Guardian:	Emergency Contact Names & Relationship:
Signature/Consent*:	
Primary Language:	Phone Number(s):

Physicians:

Primary care physician:	Emergency Phone:
	Fax:
Current Specialty physician: Specialty:	Emergency Phone:
	Fax:
Current Specialty physician: Specialty:	Emergency Phone:
	Fax:
Anticipated Primary ED:	Pharmacy:
Anticipated Tertiary Care Center:	

Diagnoses/Past Procedures/Physical Exam:

1.

Baseline physical findings:

2.

3.

Baseline vital signs:

4.

Synopsis:

Baseline neurological status:

*Consent for release of this form to health care providers

Last name:

Diagnoses/Past Procedures/Physical Exam continued:

Medications:

1.
2.
3.
4.
5.
6.

Significant baseline ancillary findings (lab, x-ray, ECG):

Prostheses/Appliances/Advanced Technology Devices:

Management Data:

Allergies: Medications/Foods to be avoided   **and why:**

1.
2.
3.

Procedures to be avoided   **and why:**

1.
2.
3.

Immunizations

Dates						Dates					
DPT						Hep B					
OPV						Varicella					
MMR						TB status					
HIB						Other					

Antibiotic prophylaxis: Indication: Medication and dose:

Common Presenting Problems/Findings With Specific Suggested Managements

Problem   Suggested Diagnostic Studies   Treatment Considerations

Comments on child, family, or other specific medical issues:

Physician/Provider Signature: **Print Name:**

CARE PLAN FOR CHILDREN WITH SPECIAL HEALTH NEEDS
-To be completed by a Health Care Provider-

	Today's Date
Child's Full Name	Date of Birth
Parent's/Guardian's Name	Telephone No. ( )
Primary Health Care Provider	Telephone No. ( )
Specialty Provider	Telephone No. ( )
Specialty Provider	Telephone No. ( )
Diagnosis(es)	
Allergies	

ROUTINE CARE

Medication To Be Given at Child Care	Schedule/Dose (When and How Much?)	Route (How?)	Reason Prescribed	Possible Side Effects

List medications given at home:

NEEDED ACCOMMODATION(S)

Describe any needed accommodation(s) the child needs in daily activities and why:

Diet or Feeding: _____

Classroom Activities: _____

Naptime/Sleeping: _____

Toileting: _____

Outdoor or Field Trips: _____

Transportation: _____

Other: _____

Additional comments: _____

_____

CH-15
MAR 05

CARE PLAN FOR CHILDREN WITH SPECIAL HEALTH NEEDS
Continued

SPECIAL EQUIPMENT / MEDICAL SUPPLIES

1. _____
2. _____
3. _____

EMERGENCY CARE

CALL PARENTS/GUARDIANS if the following symptoms are present:

_____
_____

CALL 911 (EMERGENCY MEDICAL SERVICES) if the following symptoms are present, as well as contacting the parents/guardians:

_____
_____

TAKE THESE MEASURES while waiting for parents or medical help to arrive:

_____
_____
_____

SUGGESTED SPECIAL TRAINING FOR STAFF

_____
_____
_____

Health Care Provider Signature	Date

PARENT NOTES (OPTIONAL)

_____
_____
_____

I hereby give consent for my child's health care provider or specialist to communicate with my child's child care provider or school nurse to discuss any of the information contained in this care plan.

Parent/Guardian Signature	Date

Important: *In order to ensure the health and safety of your child, it is vital that any person involved in the care of your child be aware of your child's special health needs, medication your child is taking, or needs in case of a health care emergency, and the specific actions to take regarding your child's special health needs.*

Special Health Care Plan

The special health care plan defines all members of the care team, communication guidelines (how, when, and how often), and all information on appropriately accommodating the special health concerns and needs of this child while in child care.

Name of Child: _____ **Date:** _____

Facility Name: _____

· ·

Description of condition(s): (include description of difficulties associated with each condition) _____

_____

_____

_____

Team Member Names and Titles (parents of the child are to be included)

Care Coordinator (responsible for developing and administering the Special Health Care Plan): _____

_____

_____

_____

_____

_____

_____

ⓘ   If training is necessary, then all team members will be trained.

❏ Individualized Family Service Plan **(IFSP)** attached   ❏ Individualized Education Plan **(IEP)** attached

Outside Professionals Involved   **Telephone**

Health Care Provider (MD, NP, etc.): _____   _____

Speech & Language Therapist: _____   _____

Occupational Therapist: _____   _____

Physical Therapist: _____   _____

Psychologist/Mental Health Consultant: _____   _____

Social Worker: _____   _____

Family-Child Advocate: _____   _____

Other: _____   _____

Communication

How the team will communicate (notes, communication log, phone calls, meetings, etc.):

_____

_____

How often will team communication occur: ❏ **Daily**   ❏ **Weekly**   ❏ **Monthly**   ❏ **Bi-monthly**   ❏ **Other** _____

Date and time specifics: _____

        California Childcare Health Program www.ucsfchildcarehealth.org   rev. 08/04

Specific Medical Information

❖ Medical documentation provided and attached: ❏ Yes ❏ No

❏ **Information Exchange Form** completed by health care provider is in child's file on site.

❖ Medication to be administered: ❏ Yes ❏ No

❏ **Medication Administration Form** completed by health care provider and parents are in child's file on site (including: type of medications, method, amount, time schedule, potential side effects, etc.)

Any known allergies to foods and/or medications: _____

Specific health-related needs: _____

_____

_____

_____

_____

Planned strategies to support the child's needs and any safety issues while in child care: (diapering/toileting, outdoor play, circle time, nap/sleeping, etc.) _____

_____

_____

_____

_____

_____

Plan for absences of personnel trained and responsible for health-related procedure(s): _____

_____

_____

Other (i.e., transportation, field trips, etc.): _____

_____

Special Staff Training Needs

Training monitored by: _____

1) Type (be specific): _____

Training done by: _____ Date of Training: _____

2) Type (be specific): _____

Training done by: _____ Date of Training: _____

3) Type (be specific): _____

Training done by: _____ Date of Training: _____

Equipment/Positioning

❖ Physical Therapist (PT) and/or Occupational Therapist (OT) consult provided: ❏ Yes ❏ No ❏ Not Needed

Special equipment needed/to be used: _____

_____

Positioning requirements (attach additional documentation as necessary): _____

_____

Equipment care/maintenance notes: _____

Nutrition and Feeding Needs

❏ **Nutrition and Feeding Care Plan Form** completed by team is in child's file on-site. (See for detailed requirements/needs.)

Behavior Changes (be specific when listing changes in behavior that arise as a result of the health-related condition/concerns)

_____

_____

_____

Additional Information (include any unusual episodes that might arise while in care and how the situation should be handled)

_____

_____

_____

Support Programs the Child Is Involved with Outside of Child Care

1. Name of program: _____ Contact person: _____

   Address and telephone: _____

   Frequency of attendance: _____

2. Name of program: _____ Contact person: _____

   Address and telephone: _____

   Frequency of attendance: _____

3. Name of program: _____ Contact person: _____

   Address and telephone: _____

   Frequency of attendance: _____

Emergency Procedures

❏ Special emergency and/or medical procedure required (additional documentation attached)

Emergency instructions: _____

_____

_____

Emergency contact: _____ Telephone: _____

Follow-up: Updates/Revisions

This Special Health Care Plan is to be updated/revised whenever child's health status changes or at least every _____ months as a result of the collective input from team members.

Due date for revision and team meeting: _____

California Childcare Health Program www.ucsfchildcarehealth.org rev. 08/04

SAMPLE ASTHMA ACTION PLAN

Asthma Action Plan, for Children 0–5 Years

Name _____

DOB _____

Record # _____

Health Care Provider's Name _____

Health Care Provider's Phone Number _____ Completed by _____ Date _____

Long-Term Control Medicines (Use every day to stay healthy)	How Much To Take	How Often	Other Instructions (such as spacers/masks, nebulizers)
		_____ times per day EVERY DAY	
		_____ times per day EVERY DAY	
		_____ times per day EVERY DAY	

Quick-Relief Medicines	How Much To Take	How Often	Other Instructions
		Give ONLY as needed	NOTE: If this medicine is needed often (_____ per week), call physician

GREEN ZONE

Child is WELL and has no asthma symptoms, even during active play

Prevent asthma symptoms every day
- **Give the above long-term control medicines every day**
- Avoid things that make the child's asthma worse
- ☑ Avoid tobacco smoke, ask people to smoke outside
- ☐ _____
- ☐ _____

YELLOW ZONE

Child is NOT WELL and has asthma symptoms that may incude:
- Coughing
- Wheezing
- Runny nose or other cold symptoms
- Breathing harder or faster
- Awakening due to coughing or difficulty breating
- Playing less than usual
- _____
- _____

Other symptoms that could indicate that your child is having trouble breathing may include: difficulty feeding (grunting sounds, poor sucking), changes in sleep patterns, cranky and tired, decreased appetite

CAUTION: Take action by continuing to give regular asthma medicines every day AND:
- ☐ Give _____
  _____ (include dose and frequency)

If the Child is not in the *Green Zone* and still has symptoms after 1 hour:
- ☐ Give _____
  _____ (include dose and frequency)
- ☐ Give _____
  _____ (include dose and frequency)
- ☐ Call _____

RED ZONE

Child FEELS AWFUL warning signs may incude:
- Child's wheeze, cough or difficult breathing continues or worsens, even after giving yellow zone medicines
- Child's breathing is so hard that he/she is having trouble walking/talking/eating/playing
- Child is drowsy or less alert than normal

DANGER!

Get help immediately! Call 9-1-1 if:

MEDICAL ALERT! Get help!
- ☐ Take the child to the hospital or call 9-1-1 immediately!
- ☐ Give more _____
  _____ (include dose and frequency) until you get help
- ☐ Give more _____
  _____ (include dose and frequency) until you get help

- **The child's skin is sucked in around neck and ribs or**
- **Lips and/or fingernails are grey or blue, or**
- **Child doesn't respond to you.**

Source: http://www.calasthma.org/uploads/resources/actionplanpdf.pdf. San Francisco Bay Area Regional Asthma Management Plan. http://www.rampasthma.org

Source: National Heart, Lung, and Blood Institute National Asthma Education and Prevention. *Expert Panel Report 3; Guidelines for the Diagnosis and Management of Asthma; Full Report 2007*. Bethesda, MD: NHLBI; 2007:118.

Patient Name _____ DOB _____

Asthma Action Plan, for Children 0–5 Years, *continued*

PROVIDER INSTRUCTIONS FOR ASTHMA ACTION PLAN (Children ages 0-5)

☐ **Determine the Level of Asthma severity** (see Table 1)

☐ **Fill In Medications**
Fill in medications appropriate to that level (see Table 1) and include instructions, such as "shake well before using" "use with spacer", and "rinse mouth after using".

☐ **Address Issues Related To Asthma Severity**
These can include allergens, smoke, rhinitis, sinusitis, gastro-esophaegeal reflux, sulfite sensitivity, medication interactions, and viral respiratory infections.

☐ **Fill in and Review Action Steps**
Complete the recommendations for action in the different zones, and review the whole plan with the family so they are clear on how to adjust the medications, and when to call for help.

☐ **Distribute copies of the plan**
Give the top copy of the plan to the family, the next one to school, day care, caretaker, or other involved third party as appropriate, and file the last copy in the chart.

☐ **Review Action plan Regularly (Step Up/Step Down Therapy)**
A patient who is always in the green zone for some months may be a candidate to "step down" and be reclassified to a lower level of asthma severity and treatment. A patient frequently in the yellow or red zone should be assessed to make sure inhaler technique is correct, adherence is good, environmental factors are not interfering with treatment, and alternative diagnoses have been considered. If these considerations are met, the patient should "step up" to a higher classification of asthma severity and treatment. Be sure to fill out a new asthma action plan when changes in treatment are made.

TABLE 1 SEVERITY AND MEDICATION CHART (Classification is based on meeting at least one criterion)

	Severe Persistent	Moderate Persistent	Mild Persistent	Mild Intermittent
Symptoms/Day	Consistent symptoms	Daily symptoms	> 2 days/week but < 1 time/day	≤ 2 days/week
Symptoms/Night	Frequent	> 1 night/week	> 2 nights/month	≤ 2 nights/month
Long Term Control[1]	**Preferred treatment:** • Daily *high-dose* inhaled corticosteroid **AND** • Log acting inhaled B$_2$ – agonist **AND, if needed:** • Corticosteroid tablets or syrup long term (2 mg/kg/day, generally do not exceed 60 mg per day). (Make repeated attempts to reduce systemic corticosteroids and maintain control with high-dose inhaled corticosteroids.) *Consultation With Asthma Specialist Recommended*	**Preferred treatment:** • Daily *low dose* inhaled corticosteroid and long-acting inhaled B$_2$ – agonist OR • Daily *medium-dose* inhaled corticosteroid **Alternative treatment:** • Daily *low-dose* inhaled corticosteroid and either leukotriene receptor antagonist or theophylline ...... **If needed** (particularly in patients with recurring severe exacerbations): **Preferred treatment:** • Daily *medium dose* inhaled corticosteroid and long-acting inhaled B$_2$ – agonist **Alternative treatment:** • Daily *medium-dose* inhaled corticosteroid and either leukotriene receptor antagonist or theophylline *Consultation With Asthma Specialist Recommended*	**Preferred treatment:** • Daily *low dose* inhaled corticosteroid (with nebulizer or MDI with holding chamber with or without face mask or DPI) **Alternative treatment:** • Cromolyn (nebulizer is preferred or MDI with holding chamber) **OR** • Leukotriene receptor antagonist **Note:** Initiation of long-term controller therapy should be considered if child has had more then three episodes of wheezing in the past year that lasted more than one day and affected sleep and who have risk factors for the development of asthma[2] *Consultation With Asthma Specialist Recommended*	**NO** daily medication needed.
Quick Relief[1]	**Preferred treatment:** • Inhaled short-acting B$_2$ – Agonist **Alternative treatment:** • Oral B$_2$ – agonist	**Preferred treatment:** • Inhaled short-acting B$_2$ – Agonist **Alternative treatment:** • Oral B$_2$ – agonist	**Preferred treatment:** • Inhaled short-acting B$_2$ – Agonist **Alternative treatment:** • Oral B$_2$ – agonist	**Preferred treatment:** • Inhaled short-acting B$_2$ – Agonist **Alternative treatment:** • Oral B$_2$ – agonist

[1] For infants and children use spacer or spacer AND MASK.

[2] Risk factors for the development of asthma are parental history of asthma, physician-diagnosed etopic dermatitis or two of the following: physician-diagnosed allergic rhinitis, wheezing apart from colds, peripheral blood eosinophilia. With viral respiratory infection, use bronchodilator every 4-6 hours up to 24 hours (longer with physician consult); in general no more than once every six weeks. If patient has seasonal asthma on a predictable basis, long-term anti-inflammatory therapy (inhaled corticosteroids, cromolyn) should be initiated prior to the anticipated onset of symptoms and continued through the season.

This Asthma Plan was developed by a committee facilitated by the Childhood Asthma Initiative, a program funded by the California Children and Families Commission, and the Regional Asthma Management and Prevention (RAMP) Initiative, a program of the Public Health Institute. This plan is based on the recommendations from the National Heart, Lung, and Blood Institute's. "Guidelines for the Diagnosis and Management of Asthma." NIH Publication No. 97-4051 (April 1997) and "Update on Selected Topics 2002." NIH Publication No. 02-5075 (June 2002). The information contained herein is intended for the use and convenience of physicians and other medical personnel, and may not be appropriate for use in all circumstances. Decisions to adopt any particular recommendation must be made by qualified medical personnel in light of available resources and the circumstances presented by individual patients. No entity or individual involved in the funding or development of this plan makes any warranty guarantee, express or implied, of the quality, fitness, performance or results of use of the information or products described in the plan or the Guidelines. For additional information, please contact RAMP at (510) 622-4438, http://www.rampasthma.org.

Asthma Action Plan, for Children 6 Years or Older

Name _____

DOB _____

Record # _____

Health Care Provider's Name _____

Health Care Provider's Phone Number _____ Completed by _____ Date _____

Long-Term Control Medicines (Use every day to stay healthy)	How Much To Take	How Often	Other Instructions (such as spacers/masks, nebulizers)
		_____ times per day EVERY DAY	
		_____ times per day EVERY DAY	
		_____ times per day EVERY DAY	
		_____ times per day EVERY DAY	

Quick-Relief Medicines	How Much To Take	How Often	Other Instructions
		Take ONLY as needed	NOTE: If this medicine is needed frequently, call physician to consider increasing long-term-control medications

Special instructions when I feel **good** (green), **not good** (yellow), and **awful** (red).

GREEN ZONE

I feel **good.**

(My **peak flow** is in the **GREEN** zone.)

GREEN Peak Flow My Personal Best

Prevent asthma symptoms everyday

☐ Take my long-term-control medicines (above) every day

☐ Before exercise, take _____ puffs of

_____

☐ Avoid things that make my asthma worse like:_____

_____

YELLOW ZONE

I do **not** feel **good.**

(My **peak flow** is in the **YELLOW** zone.)

My symptoms may include one or more of the following:

• Wheeze
• Tight chest
• Cough
• Shortness of breath
• Waking up at night with asthma symptoms
• Decreased ability to do usual activities
• _____
• _____

YELLOW 80% Personal Best

CAUTION: I should continue taking my long-term-control asthma medicines every day AND:

☐ Take _____

_____

If I do not feel good, or my peak flow is not in the *Green Zone* within 1 hour, then I should:

☐ Increase _____

☐ Add _____

☐ Call _____

RED ZONE

I feel **awful**:

(My **peak flow** is in the **RED** zone.)

Warning signs may include one or more of the following:

• It's getting harder and harder to breathe.
• Unable to sleep or do usual activities because of trouble breathing.

RED 50% Personal Best

Liters/Min.

Peak Flow Meter

MEDICAL ALERT! Get help!

☐ Take _____
until I get help immediately!

☐ Take _____

☐ Call _____

DANGER! Get help immediately!

Call 9-1-1 if you have trouble walking or talking due to shortness of breath or lips or fingernails are gray or blue.

Source: Adapted and reprinted with permission from the Regional Asthma Management and Prevention (RAMP) initiative, a program of the Public Health Institute. http://www.calasthma.org/uploads/resources/actionplanpdf.pdf. San Francisco Bay Area Regional Asthma Management Plan.

Source: http://www.calasthma.org/uploads/resources/actionplanpdf.pdf. San Francisco Bay Area Regional Asthma Management Plan. http://www.rampasthma.org

Source: National Heart, Lung, and Blood Institute National Asthma Education and Prevention. *Expert Panel Report 3; Guidelines for the Diagnosis and Management of Asthma; Full Report 2007.* Bethesda, MD: NHLBI; 2007:117.

Patient Name _____ DOB _____

Asthma Action Plan, for Children 6 Years or Older, *continued*

Doctor _____ Doctor's Phone Number _____ Date _____

Hospital/Emergency Department Phone Number _____

GREEN ZONE

Doing Well
- No cough, wheeze, chest tightness, or shortness of breath during the day or night
- Can do usual activities

And, if a peak flow meter is used,

Peak flow: more than _____
(80 percent or more of my best peak flow)

My best peak flow is: _____

Take these long-term-control medicines each day (include an anti-inflammatory).

Medicine	How much to take	When to take it

Identify and avoid and control the things that make your asthma worse, like (list here):

_____
_____

Before exercise, if prescribed , take: ☐ 2 or ☐ 4 puffs   5 to 60 minutes before exercise

YELLOW ZONE

ASTHMA IS GETTING WORSE.
- Cough, wheeze, chest tightness or short-ness of breath, or
- Waking at night due to asthma or
- Can do some but not all usual activities

–OR–

Peak Flow: _____ to _____
(50 to 79 percent of my best peak flow)

1 Add quick-relief medicine — and keep taking your GREEN ZONE medicine.

_____ ☐ 2 or ☐ 4 puffs every 20 minutes for up to 1 hour
(short acting B₂ agonist) ☐ Nebulizer, once

If applicable remove yourself from the thing that made your asthma worse

2 **If your symptoms (and peak flow, if used) return to GREEN ZONE after 1 hour of above treatment:**
☐ Continue monitoring to be sure you stay in the green zone

–OR –

If your symptoms (and peak flow, if used) do NOT return to GREEN ZONE after 1 hour of above treatment:

☐ Take _____ ☐ 2 or ☐ 4 puffs or ☐ Nebulizer
(short acting B₂ agonist)

☐ Add _____ _____ mg per day. For _____ (3-10) days
(oral corticosteroid)

☐ Call the doctor _____ ☐ before ☐ within _____ hours after taking the oral corticosteroid
(phone)

RED ZONE

MEDICAL ALERT
- Very short of breath, or
- Quick relief medicines have not helped, or
- Cannot do usual activies, or
- Symptoms are same or get worse after 24 hours in Yellow Zone

–OR–

Peak Flow: less than _____
(50 percent of my best peak flow)

Take this medication:

☐ _____ ☐ 4 or ☐ 6 puffs or ☐ Nebulizer
(short acting B₂ agonist)

☐ _____ _____ mg.
(oral corticosteroid)

Then call your doctor NOW. Go to the hospital or call an ambulance if:
- You are still in the RED ZONE after 15 minutes AND
- You have not reached your doctor

Danger Signs • **Trouble walking and talking due to shortness of breath**
• **Lips or figernails are blue**

- **Take** ☐ **4 or** ☐ **6 puffs of your quick-relief medication AND**
- **Go to the hospital or call for an ambulance** _____ **NOW**
(phone)

Source: National Heart,Lung, and Blood Institute. National Institutes of Health, U.S. Department of Health and Human Services. NIH Publication No 07-5251, October 2006.
Source: National Heart, Lung, and Blood Institute National Asthma Education and Prevention. *Expert Panel Report 3; Guidelines for the Diagnosis and Management of Asthma; Full Report 2007.*
Bethesda, MD: NHLBl; 2007:119.

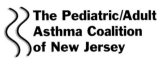

**The Pediatric/Adult
Asthma Coalition
of New Jersey**

"Your Pathway to Asthma Control"
Original PACNJ approved Plan available at
www.pacnj.org

Asthma Treatment Plan
Patient/Parent Instructions

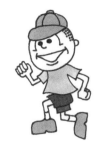

The **PACNJ Asthma Treatment Plan** is designed to help everyone understand the steps necessary for the individual patient to achieve the goal of controlled asthma.

1. Patients/Parents/Guardians: *Before taking this form to your Health Care Provider:*
Complete the top left section with:

- Patient's name
- Patient's date of birth
- Patient's doctor's name & phone number
- Parent/Guardian's name & phone number
- An Emergency Contact person's name & phone number

2. Your Health Care Provider will:
Complete the following areas:
- The effective date of this plan
- The medicine information for the Healthy, Caution and Emergency sections
- Your Health Care Provider will check the box next to the medication and circle how much and how often to take it
- Your Health Care Provider may check **"OTHER"** and:
    - ❖ **Write in asthma medications not listed on the form**
    - ❖ **Write in additional medications that will control your asthma**
    - ❖ **Write in generic medications in place of the name brand on the form**
- Together you and your Health Care Provider will decide what asthma treatment is best for you or your child to follow

3. Patients/Parents/Guardians & Health Care Providers together:
Discuss and then complete the following areas:
- Patient's peak flow range in the Healthy, Caution and Emergency sections on the left side of the form
- Patient's asthma triggers on the right side of the form
- <u>For Minors Only</u> section at the bottom of the form: Discuss your child's ability to self-administer the inhaled medications, check the appropriate box, and then both you and your Health Care Provider must sign and date the form

4. Parents/Guardians: *After completing the form with your Health Care Provider:*
- Make copies of the Asthma Treatment Plan and give the signed original to your child's school nurse or child care provider
- Keep a copy easily available at home to help manage your child's asthma
- Give copies of the Asthma Treatment Plan to everyone who provides care for your child, for example: babysitters, before/after school program staff, coaches, scout leaders

This Asthma Treatment Plan is meant to assist, not replace, the clinical decision-making required to meet individual patient needs. Not all asthma medications are listed and the generic names are not listed.

The Pediatric/Adult Asthma Coalition of New Jersey, sponsored by the American Lung Association of New Jersey, and this publication are supported by a grant from the New Jersey Department of Health and Senior Services (NJDHSS), with funds provided by the U.S. Centers for Disease Control and Prevention (USCDCP) under Cooperative Agreement 5U59EH000206-2. Its contents are solely the responsibility of the authors and do not necessarily represent the official views of the NJDHSS or the USCDCP. Although this document has been funded wholly or in part by the United States Environmental Protection Agency under Agreements XA97256707-1, XA98284401-3 and XA97250908-0 to the American Lung Association of New Jersey, it has not gone through the Agency's publications review process and therefore, may not necessarily reflect the views of the Agency and no official endorsement should be inferred. Information in this publication is not intended to diagnose health problems or take the place of medical advice. For asthma or any medical condition, seek medical advice from your child's or your health care professional.

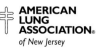

**AMERICAN
LUNG
ASSOCIATION**®
of New Jersey

Asthma Treatment Plan

(This asthma action plan meets NJ Law N.J.S.A. 18A:40-12.8) (Physician's Orders)

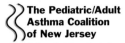

The Pediatric/Adult Asthma Coalition of New Jersey

"Your Pathway to Asthma Control"
Original PACNJ approved Plan available at
www.pacnj.org

Sponsored by
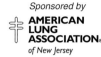
AMERICAN LUNG ASSOCIATION®
of New Jersey

NEW JERSEY DEPARTMENT OF HEALTH & SENIOR SERVICES

(Please Print)

Name	Date of Birth	Effective Date

Doctor	Parent/Guardian (if applicable)	Emergency Contact

Phone	Phone	Phone

HEALTHY ▕▐▐▌➡

You have _all_ of these:
• Breathing is good
• No cough or wheeze
• Sleep through the night
• Can work, exercise, and play

And/Or Peak flow above _____

Take daily medicine(s). All metered dose inhalers (MDI) to be used with spacers.

MEDICINE	HOW MUCH to take and HOW OFTEN to take it
☐ Advair® ☐ 100, ☐ 250, ☐ 500	. . . . .1 inhalation twice a day
☐ Advair® HFA ☐ 45, ☐ 115, ☐ 230	. . . . . . .2 puffs MDI twice a day
☐ Asmanex® Twisthaler® ☐ 110, ☐ 220	. . . . . .☐ 1, ☐ 2 inhalations a day
☐ Flovent® ☐ 44, ☐ 110, ☐ 220	. . . . .2 inhalations twice a day
☐ Flovent® Diskus® 50 mcg	. . . . .1 inhalation twice a day
☐ Pulmicort Flexhaler® ☐ 90, ☐ 180	. . . . .☐ 1, ☐ 2 inhalations ☐ once or ☐ twice a day
☐ Pulmicort Respules® ☐ 0.25, ☐ 0.5, ☐ 1.0	.1 unit nebulized ☐ once or ☐ twice a day
☐ Qvar® ☐ 40, ☐ 80	. . . . .2 inhalations twice a day
☐ Singulair ☐ 4, ☐ 5, ☐ 10 mg	. . . . .1 tablet daily
☐ Symbicort® ☐ 80, ☐ 160	. . . . .2 puffs MDI twice a day
☐ Other	
☐ None	

Remember to rinse your mouth after taking inhaled medicine.

If exercise triggers your asthma, take this medicine_____ _____minutes before exercise.

CAUTION ▕▐▐▌➡

You have _any_ of these:
• Exposure to known trigger
• Cough
• Mild wheeze
• Tight chest
• Coughing at night
• Other:_____

And/Or Peak flow from_____ to_____

Continue daily medicine(s) and add fast-acting medicine(s).

MEDICINE	HOW MUCH to take and HOW OFTEN to take it
☐ Accuneb® ☐ 0.63, ☐ 1.25 mg	. . . . .1 unit nebulized every 4 hours as needed
☐ Albuterol ☐ 1.25, ☐ 2.5 mg	. . . . .1 unit nebulized every 4 hours as needed
☐ Albuterol ☐ Pro-Air ☐ Proventil®	. . . . . .2 puffs MDI every 4 hours as needed
☐ Ventolin® ☐ Maxair ☐ Xopenex®	. . . . . .2 puffs MDI every 4 hours as needed
☐ Xopenex® ☐ 0.31, ☐ 0.63, ☐ 1.25 mg	. .1 unit nebulized every 4 hours as needed
☐ Increase the dose of, or add:	

➡ **If fast-acting medicine is needed more than 2 times a week, except before exercise, then call your doctor.**

EMERGENCY ▕▐▐▌➡

Your asthma is getting worse fast:
• Fast-acting medicine did not help within 15-20 minutes
• Breathing is hard and fast
• Nose opens wide
• Ribs show
• Trouble walking and talking
• Lips blue • Fingernails blue

And/Or Peak flow below _____

Take these medicines NOW and call 911.
Asthma can be a life-threatening illness. Do not wait!

☐ Accuneb® ☐ 0.63, ☐ 1.25 mg	. . . . .1 unit nebulized every 20 minutes
☐ Albuterol ☐ 1.25, ☐ 2.5 mg	. . . . .1 unit nebulized every 20 minutes
☐ Albuterol ☐ Pro-Air ☐ Proventil®	. . . . . .2 puffs MDI every 20 minutes
☐ Ventolin® ☐ Maxair ☐ Xopenex®	. . . . . .2 puffs MDI every 20 minutes
☐ Xopenex® ☐ 0.31, ☐ 0.63, ☐ 1.25 mg	. .1 unit nebulized every 20 minutes
☐ Other	

Triggers
Check all items that trigger patient's asthma:

❏ Chalk dust
❏ Cigarette Smoke & second hand smoke
❏ Colds/Flu
❏ Dust mites, dust, stuffed animals, carpet
❏ Exercise
❏ Mold
❏ Ozone alert days
❏ Pests - rodents & cockroaches
❏ Pets - animal dander
❏ Plants, flowers, cut grass, pollen
❏ Strong odors, perfumes, cleaning products, scented products
❏ Sudden temperature change
❏ Wood Smoke
❏ Foods:
_____
_____
_____

❏ Other:
_____
_____
_____
_____

This asthma treatment plan is meant to assist, not replace, the clinical decision-making required to meet individual patient needs.

The Pediatric/Adult Asthma Coalition of New Jersey, sponsored by the American Lung Association of New Jersey, and this publication are supported by a grant from the New Jersey Department of Health and Senior Services (NJDHSS), with funds provided by the U.S. Centers for Disease Control and Prevention (USCDCP) under Cooperative Agreement 5U59EH000206-2. Its contents are solely the responsibility of the authors and do not necessarily represent the official views of the NJDHSS or the USCDCP.

Although this document has been funded wholly or in part by the United States Environmental Protection Agency under Agreements XA96284401-4 and XA97256707-1 to the American Lung Association of New Jersey, it has not gone through the Agency's publications review process and therefore, may not necessarily reflect the views of the Agency and no official endorsement should be inferred.

EFFECTIVE MARCH 2008
Permission to reproduce blank form
Approved by the New Jersey Thoracic Society

FOR MINORS ONLY:

☐ This student is capable and has been instructed in the proper method of self-administering of the inhaled medications named above in accordance with NJ Law.

☐ This student is _not_ approved to self-medicate.

PHYSICIAN/APN/PA SIGNATURE_____ DATE_____

PARENT/GUARDIAN SIGNATURE_____

PHYSICIAN STAMP

Make a copy for patient and for physician file. For children under 18, send original to school nurse or child care provider.

When Should Students With Asthma or Allergies Carry and Self-Administer Emergency Medications at School?

Guidance for Health Care Providers Who Prescribe Emergency Medications

Physicians and others authorized to prescribe medications, working together with parents and school nurses, should consider the list of factors below in determining when to entrust and encourage a student with diagnosed asthma and/or anaphylaxis to carry and self-administer prescribed emergency medications at school.

Most students can better manage their asthma or allergies and can more safely respond to symptoms if they carry and self-administer their life saving medications at school. **Each student should have a personal asthma/allergy management plan on file at school that addresses carrying and self-administering emergency medications**. If carrying medications is not initially deemed appropriate for a student, then his/her asthma/allergy management plan should include action steps for developing the necessary skills or behaviors that would lead to this goal. All schools need to abide by state laws and policies related to permitting students to carry and self-administer asthma inhalers and epinephrine auto-injectors.

Health care providers should assess student, family, school, and community factors in determining when a student should carry and self-administer life saving medications. **Health care providers should communicate their recommendation to the parent/guardian and the school**, and maintain communication with the school, especially the school nurse. Assessment of the factors below should help to establish a profile that guides the decision; however, responses will not generate a "score" that clearly differentiates students who would be successful.

Student factors:

- Desire to carry and self-administer
- Appropriate age, maturity, or developmental level
- Ability to identify signs and symptoms of asthma and/or anaphylaxis
- Knowledge of proper medication use in response to signs/symptoms
- Ability to use correct technique in administering medication
- Knowledge about medication side effects and what to report
- Willingness to comply with school's rules about use of medicine at school, for example:
  - Keeping one's bronchodilator inhaler and/or auto-injectable epinephrine with him/her at all times;
  - Notifying a responsible adult (e.g., teacher, nurse, coach, playground assistant) during the day when a bronchodilator inhaler is used and *immediately* when auto-injectable epinephrine is used;
  - Not sharing medication with other students or leaving it unattended;
  - Not using bronchodilator inhaler or auto-injectable epinephrine for any other use than what is intended;
- Responsible carrying and self-administering medicine at school in the past (e.g. while attending a previous school or during an after-school program).

NOTE: Although past asthma history is not a sure predictor of future asthma episodes, those children with a history of asthma symptoms and episodes might benefit the most from carrying and self-administering emergency medications at school. It may be useful to consider the following.

- Frequency and location of past sudden onsets
- Presence of triggers at school
- Frequency of past hospitalizations or emergency department visits due to asthma

Parent/guardian factors:

- Desire for the student to self-carry and self-administer
- Awareness of school medication policies and parental responsibilities
- Commitment to making sure the student has the needed medication with them, medications are refilled when needed, back-up medications are provided, and medication use at school is monitored through collaborative effort between the parent/guardian and the school team

School and community factors:

In making the assessment of when a student should carry and self-administer emergency medicines, it can be useful to factor in available school resources and adherence to policies aimed at providing students with a safe environment for taking medicines. Such factors include:

- Presence of a full-time school nurse or health assistant in the school all day every day
- Availability of trained staff to administer medications to students who do not self-carry and to those who do (in case student looses or is unable to properly take his/her medication); to monitor administration of medications by students who do self-carry
- Provision for safe storage and easy, immediate access to students' medications for both those who do not self-carry and for access to back-up medicine for those who do
- Close proximity of stored medicine in relationship to student's classroom and playing fields
- Availability of medication and trained staff for off-campus activities
- Communication systems in school (intercom, walkie-talkie, cell phones, pagers) to contact appropriate staff in case of a medical emergency
- Past history of appropriately dealing with asthma and/or anaphylaxis episodes by school staff
- Provision of opportunities for asthma and anaphylaxis basic training for school staff (including after-school coaches and bus drivers)

NOTE: The goal is for all students to eventually carry and self-administer their medications. However, on one hand, if a school has adequate resources and adheres to policies that promote safe and appropriate administration of life-saving medications by staff, there may be less relative benefit for younger, less mature students in this school to carry and self-administer their medication. On the other hand, if sufficient resources and supportive policies are NOT in place at school, it may be prudent to assign greater weight to student and family factors in determining when a student should self-carry.

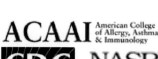

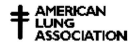
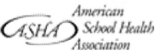
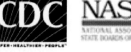
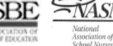

This guidance sheet was developed as a partnership activity facilitated by the NAEPP, coordinated by the NHLBI of the NIH/DHHS

March 2005

Caring for Our Children:
National Health and Safety Performance Standards

Adaptive Equipment for Children With Special Needs

Physical Therapy/Occupational Therapy Equipment

Infants, Ages 0-2

Equipment
Floor mats, 2-3-inch of varying firmness
Therapy balls of varying sizes
Wedges: 4, 6, 8 and 12-inch
Inflatable mattress
Air compressor (for inflatables)
Therapy rolls and half rolls of varying sizes
Nesting benches, varying heights
Wooden weighted pushcart
Toddler swing
Floor mirror

Feeding
Bottle straws
Cut-out cups
Bottle holders
Built-up handled utensils
Scoop bowls
Coated spoons

Toys
Books
Mirror
Ring stack
Container toys
Pegboard
Rattles
Squeeze toys
Tracking toys
Toys for pushing, swiping, cause and effect
Form boards
Large beads
Large crayons

Pre-K, Ages 2-5

Equipment
Floor mats, 2-3-inch of varying firmness
Therapy balls: 16, 20, 24 and 37-inch diameter
Nesting benches
Therapy rolls: 8, 10 and 12-inch diameter
Steps
Floor mirrors
Climbing equipment
Small chair and table
Scooter board
Suspended equipment (see also Adaptive Physical
    Education Equipment, Balance/Gross Motor
    Coordination)
Walkers, sidelyers, proneboards, adapted chairs

Toys
Easel
Tricycles
Ride-on scooters
Wagon
Wooden push cart
Manipulative toys (puzzles, beads, pegs and pegboard,
    nesting toys, etc.)
Fastening boards (zippers, snaps, laces, etc.)
Paper, crayons, chalk, markers
Sand/water table
Play-Doh or clay
Target activities (beanbags, ring toss)
Playground balls (see under Adaptive Physical
Education Equipment, Eye-Hand Coordination)

Adaptive Equipment for Children With Special Needs

Speech and Language Development

Infants, Ages 0-2

Equipment
Mirrors, wall and hand-held
Assorted spoons, cups, bowls, plates
Mats and sheets
Preston feeding chairs
High chair

Toys
Dolls (soft with large features and feeding equipment)
Rattles (noisemakers and easy to grasp)
Manipulative toys (for pulling, pushing,
    shaking, cause and effect)
Assorted picture books (large pictures, one-a-page)
Building blocks
Balls/belts
Telephone
Stacking rings
Shape sorters
Xylophone
Drum

Assessments and Books
Small Wonder Activity Kit
Pre-Feeding Skills by Suzanne Morris
Parent-Infant Communication
Bayley Scales of Infant Development
Movement Assessment in Infants by S. Harris
    and L. Chandler
RIDES
HAWAII HELP
Early Learning Accomplishments
    Profile and Kit (Kaplan)
Rosetti Infant/Toddler Language Scale

Pre-K, Ages 2-5

Equipment
Mirrors, wall and hand-held
Tongue depressors
Penlight
Stopwatch
Tape recorder and tapes
Toothettes
Horns and Whistles

Toys
Dolls (with movable parts and removable clothing)
Manipulative toys (cars and toys for pushing, stack-
    ing, cause and effect)
Building blocks
Dollhouse
Pretend play items (dress-up clothes, dishes, sink,
    food, telephone)
Play-Doh or clay
Puzzles (individual pieces or minimal interlocking
    parts)
Picture cards (nouns, actions, etc.)
Puppets
Animals
Storybooks with simple plot lines (large pictures and
    few, if any, words)

Assessments and books
Clinical evaluation of Language Fundamentals –
    Pre-School
Sequenced Inventory of Communication
Test of Auditory Comprehension of Language
Goldman Fristore Test of Articulation
Pre-School Language Assessment Inventory
Assessment of Phonological Processes
Expressive and Receptive One-Word Picture
Vocabulary Tests

Caring for Our Children:
National Health and Safety Performance Standards

Adaptive Equipment for Children With Special Needs

Adaptive Physical Education Equipment

Pre-K, Ages 2-5

Balance/Gross Motor Coordination
Incline mat
Balance beams, 4 and 12-inch wide
Floor mats, 2-inch
Bolsters
Rocking platforms
Scooters (sit-on type)
Tunnel (accordion style)
Training stairs
Hurdles, adjustable height

Eye-Hand Coordination
Balls (to hit, throw, and catch)
Beanbags and Target
Hula hoops
Lightweight paddles/rackets
Lightweight bats
Traffic cones
Batting Tees
Beachballs

Eye-Foot Coordination
Balls for kicking
Foot placement ladder
Footprints or "stepping stones"
Horizontal ladder

Reprinted with permission. American Academy of Pediatrics, American Public Health Association, National Resource Center for Health and Safety in Child Care and Early Education. *Caring for Our Children: National Health and Safety Performance Standards: Guidelines for Out-of-Home Child Care Programs.* 2nd ed. Elk Grove Village, IL: American Academy of Pediatrics; 2002.

Elements of a Do-Not-Resuscitate Plan for Schools

The **elements** of a do-not-resuscitate (DNR) plan should include
- Development of a district policy on the care of the child with a DNR order
- Liability protection for those involved in implementing the DNR plan
- Documentation that confirms the DNR is active and verifiable by all responding parties
- Special consideration to meeting child and family needs, as well as the needs of the students and staff
- A process for ensuring the privacy of the event so that students and staff, other than those designated, are removed from the scene
- Involvement of the child's clinician in all aspects of planning
- Reconciliation of all state statutes including pronouncement, medical examiner involvement, and emergency medical services (EMS)/911 limitations
- Involvement of the local EMS/911 and an agreement on what type of care that EMS/911 is able to provide in this situation (This needs to be outlined in the Individual Health Care Plan.)
- A process for conveying the plan to staff
- A plan for the school community to deal with the loss

The **Individual Health Care Plan** outlines the child's individual needs and provides the structure for the staff to follow in the event of a cardiac or respiratory arrest. Elements of the plan include
- Periodic review to ensure that the DNR is still active and documentation is available at all times
- How the child will be moved to the health room or other designated area if serious distress or death should occur at another location in the school
- Identification of designated staff (and backup/substitutes) who will be involved in the event
- Process for notification of EMS/911
- The comfort measures that should be given to the child
- Protocols for notification of the family
- Protocols for when the child has died in school prior to EMS/911 arrival
- The designated clinician who will do the pronouncement of death (physician, nurse practitioner, or physician assistant)
- How the deceased will be removed from the school (This may involve planning with the family's designated funeral home and include such factors as type of vehicle, where it will park, who will clear the corridors, and what kind of stretcher or other method of transport will be used.)

AMERICANS WITH DISABILITIES ACT

COMMONLY ASKED QUESTIONS RELATED TO GIVING MEDICINE IN CHILD CARE

The Americans with Disabilities Act (ADA), passed July 26, 1990 as Public Law 101-336 (42 U.S.C. Sec. 12101 *et seq.*), became effective on January 26, 1992. The ADA requires that child care provider/directors not discriminate against persons with disabilities on the basis of disability, that is, that they provide children and parent/guardians with disabilities with an equal opportunity to participate in child care programs and services. Child care facilities must make reasonable modifications to their policies and practices, such as giving medicine, to integrate children with disabilities.

1. Q: Does the Americans with Disabilities Act – or "ADA" – apply to child care centers? What about family child care homes?

A: Yes. Almost all child care facilities, even small, home-based centers regardless of size or number of employees, must comply with title III of the ADA. Child care services provided by government agencies must comply with title II. The exception is child care centers that are actually run by religious entities such as churches, mosques, or synagogues. Activities controlled by religious organizations are not covered by title III.

2. Q: Our facility has a policy that we will not give medication to any child. Can I refuse to give medication to a child with a disability?

A: No. In some circumstances, it may be necessary to give medication to a child with a disability in order to make a program accessible to that child. Disabilities include any physical or mental impairment that substantially limits one or more major life activities including asthma, diabetes, seizure disorders, or attention deficit hyperactivity disorder (ADHD).

3. Q: What about children who have severe, sometimes life-threatening allergies to bee stings or certain foods? Do we have to take them?

A: Generally, yes. Children cannot be excluded on the sole basis that they have been identified as having severe allergies to bee stings or certain foods. A child care facility needs to be prepared to take appropriate steps in the event of an allergic reaction, such as administering a medicine called "epinephrine" that will be provided in advance by the child's parents or guardians.

4. Q: What about children with diabetes? Do we have to admit them to our program? If we do, do we have to test their blood sugar levels?

A: Generally, yes. Children with diabetes should not be excluded from the program on the basis of their diabetes. Providers should obtain written authorization from the child's parents or guardians and physician and follow their directions for simple diabetes-related care. In most instances, they will authorize the provider to monitor the child's blood sugar – or "blood glucose". The child's parents or guardians are responsible for providing all appropriate testing equipment, training, and special food necessary for the child.

5. Q: What about children with asthma? Do we have to admit them to our program?

A: Generally, yes. Children with asthma should not be excluded from the program on the basis of their medical condition. Providers should obtain written authorization from the child's parents or guardians and physician and follow their directions for asthma care.

6. Q: Are there any reference books or video tapes that might help me further understand the obligations of child care providers under title III?

A: Yes, the Arc published *All Kids Count: Child Care and the ADA*, which addresses the ADA's obligations of child care providers. Copies are available by calling **1-800-433-5255.** For general information child care providers may call the Department of Justice Information Line at **1-800-514-0301.**

Source: The ADA Home Page: www.usdoj.gov/crt/ada/adahom1.htm

CHILD CARE LAW CENTER

221 PINE STREET | 3RD FLOOR | SAN FRANCISCO, CA 94104 | V 415.394.7144 | F 415.394.7140
WWW.CHILDCARELAW.ORG | INFO@CHILDCARELAW.ORG

Questions and Answers: IDEA & Child Care

1. What is the IDEA?

The Individuals with Disabilities Education Act (IDEA) guarantees children with disabilities the same access to education as children who do not have disabilities.[1] In 1975, Congress passed the IDEA in response to frequent discrimination against children with disabilities in public school systems. All states must meet the minimum *federal* IDEA standards regarding the educational rights of children with disabilities. However, *state* laws can expand these rights.

2. Who is eligible for services under the IDEA?

Children ages 0 to 21 with certain disabilities are eligible.

- *Infants and Toddlers* – are eligible for Early Intervention (EI) services under the IDEA. EI services may be necessary if a child is experiencing developmental delays or has a diagnosed physical or mental condition which has a high probability of resulting in developmental delay.[2] Some states have created a third eligibility category of children at-risk of developmental delays.[3]

- *School-age and Children Attending Preschool* – are eligible if found to have mental retardation, hearing impairments, speech or language impairments, visual impairments, serious emotional disturbance, orthopedic impairments, autism, traumatic brain injury, other health impairments, or specific learning disabilities, which as a result need special education and related services.[4]

3. How do families apply?

If a parent feels her child is eligible for services under the IDEA, she should contact her local school district or EI agency. Local educational agencies (LEA) have an obligation under federal law to "actively and systematically seek out" all persons aged 3 to 21 who would be eligible for special education.[5] The lead agency for EI services has a similar "child find" obligation for infants and toddlers.[6] Child care providers can refer children they think may be eligible, although the family must consent in writing to an assessment.

4. What is an IEP?

- An Individualized Educational Program (IEP) is an agreement that outlines a child's special education and related services.[7] An IEP is for preschool (ages 3 to 5) and school-age children.

- A team consisting of parents,[8] regular and special education teachers, a representative from the LEA, and anyone else the parent or local school district feel should be present, formulate the IEP at a collaborative meeting.[9]

- The IEP must include the child's present levels of performance, measurable annual goals, and the child's special education and related services.[10] If a child does not participate in the regular classroom or in general nonacademic and extracurricular activities, the IEP must explain why and list supports and program modifications to allow participation in the general classroom.[11] A parent must provide written consent to the services to be provided.[12]

- The team reviews the IEP at least annually, or when either a parent or a teacher request a meeting for a new assessment, lack of anticipated progress by the child, or other matters.[13]

June 15, 2009

5. **What is an IFSP?**
   - An Individualized Family Service Program (IFSP) is very similar to an IEP, but an IFSP is for EI children, ages 0 to 3.
   - An IFSP may include the infant/toddler's present levels of development, the major expected outcomes for the infant/toddler and her family, the specific EI services necessary to meet the needs of the infant/toddler and her family, the natural environments in which the services will be carried out, and steps to help the infant/toddler transition to preschool or other services.[14] A parent must provide written consent to the services to be provided.[15]
   - An IFSP is evaluated annually and is reviewed at least every 6 months or more frequently if the infant/toddler or family needs it.[16]

6. **What role can child care providers play in the IEP/IFSP process?**

   At the discretion of the parent or agency, other individuals with "knowledge or special expertise regarding the child,"[17] (IEP) or "as appropriate, persons who will be providing services to the child or family"[18] (IFSP) may participate in the IEP or IFSP meeting and planning. This could include child care providers. Child care providers can give input on services or technology that would enable the child to participate in their program.

7. **What placement can families and children obtain under the IDEA?**
   - The IDEA is designed to guarantee children with disabilities of all ages the opportunity to participate, learn, interact, and succeed in the school setting.
   - Children with disabilities in school are assured a *Free Appropriate Public Education* (FAPE). FAPE is not tied to funding and must be based on the child's educational need.[19] Placement is based on the child's individual needs and skills as outlined on her IEP.[20]
   - Inclusion is an important goal of the IDEA. Also, for *preschool* and *school-age children* with disabilities, the IDEA requires that they be placed in the *Least Restrictive*

   Environment (LRE).[21] LRE applies to extracurricular and nonacademic activities as well,[22] which can include child care.
   - *EI (ages 0 to 3)* has a "*Natural Environment*" requirement similar to the LRE.[23] A "natural environment" includes a child's home, "community settings in which children without disabilities participate,"[24] and "settings that are natural or normal for the child's age peers who have no disabilities,"[25] such as child care.

8. **What related services can families and children obtain under the IDEA?**

   Families and children can receive any service that is necessary to help a child benefit from her special education program.[26] All services under the IDEA for children ages 3 to 21 are free[27] and based on each child's educational need, not the child's disability.[28] Some examples of these services are transportation, speech pathology, psychological services, physical and occupational therapy, counseling services, and school health services. For children receiving EI services, some states charge fees based on a sliding scale and/or require access to public/private insurance.[29]

9. **Can a family get child care or afterschool care through their IEP?**
   - Children with disabilities, *from ages 3 to 5*, may receive preschool or child care services as part of their IEP. It is also possible to include consultation services between the therapists working with a child and the child's preschool or child care programs in an IEP. The IDEA makes grants available to states to extend special education services to eligible preschool aged children.[30] Some school districts may try to limit reimbursement for placement in private preschools, but this is not allowed if the placement results from the IEP.[31]
   - If afterschool care or extended day is a related service that is necessary for a *school-age child* to benefit from her special education, then a family could receive afterschool care through an IEP.[32] The related service must be connected to the child's education and needs, not family or

other issues, *except* in the case of EI where a family's needs and strengths as well as the child's are expressly considered.[33]

- A portion of the cost of child care may be paid for as part of an IFSP.[35] For example, where a child has socialization with typically developing children as a goal in his/her IFSP, the state agency can pay for the time in child care when the child is receiving this support.

10. What assistive technology is available to child care providers for children with disabilities under the IDEA?

- Assistive technology means any equipment, off-the-shelf or customized, used to increase, maintain, or improve the functional capacities of children with disabilities.[36] Some examples of assistive technology are computers, transportation aids, glasses, and hearing aids.

- If assistive technology helps a student benefit from her special education placement, including child care, then the technology is guaranteed by the school

district.[37] Parents do not have to pay for the equipment.[38]

- The need for assistive technology must be considered in every child's IEP,[39] and it is an EI[40] service that must be considered in the IFSP process. If the IEP team decides that the child needs access to those devices in non-school settings, such as child care, in order to achieve FAPE, the LEA must allow the child to use a school-purchased assistive technology device at home or in other settings.[41]

11. What rights do parents have if the school district denies a child services or a parent does not like her child's placement?

Parents or the child's representative have the right to mediation and/or a due process hearing if they disagree with their child's IEP or on any matter relating to the child's evaluation, placement, and services under the IDEA.[42] See the resource box for agencies you can contact about more information or assistance.

Useful Resources

- **Call the Child Care Law Center** at **(415) 394-7144** if you would like information about child care issues. We are a national and California child care support center for legal services programs. The following are some of our legal services:
  - Answer legal questions regarding child care on Monday and Thursday from 12p.m. to 3p.m.
  - Write many useful legal and policy publications. Visit our website at www.childcarelaw.org.
  - Conduct trainings for parents, teachers, community agencies, and others on the Americans with Disabilities Act and other disability laws.
- **Call the National Disability Rights Network**, a national voluntary membership organization for the federally mandated nationwide network of disability rights agencies, protection and advocacy systems, and client assistance programs, at **(202) 408-9514** or visit their website at www.napas.org to find out where the office is nearest you.
- **Contact the Parent Training and Information Centers and Community Groups**, which provide training and information to parents of infants, toddlers, school-aged children, and young adults with disabilities, and the professionals who work with their families in your state. To reach the parent center in your state, call the **Technical Assistance Alliance for Parent Centers (the Alliance)** at **(888) 248-0822** or visit their website at www.taalliance.org.
- **Call Disability Rights Education & Defense Fund (DREDF)**, a national law and policy center dedicated to protecting and advancing the civil rights of people with disabilities, at **(510)644-2555** or visit their website at www.dredf.org.
- **Contact Easter Seals Disability Services,** a national non-profit that provides both resources and inclusive child care services. A list of centers and services can be found at their website: http://www.easterseals.com.

This document is intended to provide general information about the topic covered. It is believed to be current and accurate as of June 2009, but the law changes often. This document is made available with the understanding that it does not render legal or other professional advice. If you need legal advice, you should seek the services of a competent attorney.

Endnotes

[1] 20 U.S.C. § 1400 et. seq.

[2] 20 U.S.C. § 1432(5).

[3] 20 U.S.C. § 1432(5)(B).

[4] 20 U.S.C. § 1401(3); see also 34 C.F.R. § 300.7(a)(1) (further specifying eligibility criteria for special education including multiply handicapped).

[5] 20 U.S.C. § 1412(a)(3).

[6] 20 U.S.C. § 1435(a)(5).

[7] 20 U.S.C. § 1414(d) (IEP); 20 U.S.C. § 1436 (IFSP).

[8] Agencies must take extra steps to include parents if they cannot attend, such as enabling them to participate via conference call. 34 C.F.R. § 300.345.

[9] 20 U.S.C. § 1414(d)(1)(B).

[10] 20 U.S.C. § 1414(d)(A).

[11] 20 U.S.C. § 1414(d)(1)(A)(iv).

[12] 20 U.S.C. § 1436(e).

[13] 20 U.S.C. § 1414(d)(4).

[14] 20 U.S.C. § 1436(d).

[15] 20 U.S.C. § 1436(e)

[16] 20 U.S.C. § 1436(b).

[17] 20 U.S.C. § 1414(d)(B).

[18] 34 C.F.R. § 303.343(a)(1).

[19] 20 U.S.C. § 1412(a)(1); 34 C.F.R. § 300.103.

[20] 20 U.S.C. § 1414(d)(3)(A).

[21] 20 U.S.C. § 1412(a)(5).

[22] 20 U.S.C. § 1414(d)(1)(A)(iii).

[23] 20 U.S.C. § 1432(4)(G).

[24] Id.

[25] 34 C.F.R. § 303.18.

[26] 20 U.S.C. § 1414(d)(1).

[27] 20 U.S.C. § 1401(9).

[28] 20 U.S.C. § 1412(a)(1); 34 C.F.R. § 300.103.

[29] INSERT CITE

[30] 20 U.S.C. § 1419.

[31] Id. § 1412(a)(10)(B); see also 34 C.F.R. § 300, App. B.

[32] 20 U.S.C. § 1401(26).

[33] 20 U.S.C. §§ 1436(a).

[35] 20 U.S.C. § 1436(d).

[36] 20 U.S.C. § 1401(1).

[37] 20 U.S.C. § 1412(a)(12)(B)(i).

[38] Id.

[39] 20 U.S.C. § 1414(d)(3)(B)(v).

[40] 34 C.F.R. § 303.12(d)(1).

[41] 34 C.F.R. § 300.105(b).

[42] 20 U.S.C. § 1415(b).

This publication, *Questions and Answers: IDEA and Child Care*, is reprinted with permission from Child Care Law Center. More information about CCLC is available at www.childcarelaw.org.

Choosing Quality Child Care: What's Best for Your Family?

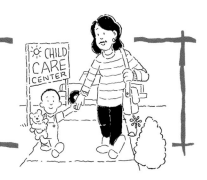

Finding high-quality child care is very important, but not always easy. Your choice will play a key role in your child's health and development. The following information may help you in your search for the child care options that are best for your family.

Types of child care

Center-based care

Center-based care has many names—child care center, preschool, nursery school, child development program, or learning center. Center-based care also may have different sponsors, including churches, schools, colleges, universities, hospitals, social service agencies, Head Start, independent owners and businesses, and employers.

Things to discuss

Before choosing a center, talk with the staff about the following:
- **Hours.** When is the center open? What if you are late in picking up your child? How are vacations and holidays scheduled?
- **Licensing/accreditation.** Is the center licensed or registered with the appropriate local government agencies? Are there any outstanding violations? Is the program currently accredited or in the process of becoming accredited?
- **Inspections/consultations.** Is there a qualified health professional, such as a doctor or nurse, for the program? (The national standard recommends that center-based infant-toddler programs should be visited by a health professional at least once a month, and all other child care programs should be visited at least once every 3 months.)
- **Visiting policy.** Can you visit the center before your child is enrolled? If your child is enrolled, can you visit the center anytime it is open? Can you see all the areas that your child will use? Are visitors screened or is their identification checked, so that only approved adults can visit the center and pick up children?
- **Experience and training.** What education, training, and experience do the staff have? What type of additional training has the staff had during the past year? Do outside experts provide training?
- **Adequate staffing.** Are there enough trained adults available on a regular basis? What happens if staff are ill or on vacation? Are children supervised by sight and sound at all times, even when they are sleeping?

  Do the child-staff ratios and the size of the groups of children fall within nationally recognized standards? For example, in a room with 4 children aged 13 to 30 months, there should be 1 trained caregiver. In a room with 5 to 8 children aged 13 to 30 months, there should be 2 trained caregivers. There should be no more than 8 children aged 13 to 30 months in a room. (See chart)

Age	Child-Staff Ratio*	Maximum Group Size*
Birth–12 months	3:1	6
13–30 months	4:1	8
31–35 months	5:1	10
3-year-olds	7:1	14
4–5-year-olds	8:1	16
6–8-year-olds	10:1	20
9–12-year-olds	12:1	24

*As recommended by the AAP. See *Caring for Our Children* listed in "Resources."

- **Health standards.** Do children need a medical exam before they can enroll? Have staff been checked by a doctor to be sure that they are healthy? What are the policies when children are mildly ill?
- **Quality.** Are children cared for in small groups? Are activities proper for their age group? Is there a daily schedule? Is there daily indoor and outdoor play time? Can children watch TV and if so, what is watched and for how long?
- **Policies.** Check the center's written policies. What is the discipline policy? Do the children go on outings? If they travel by car, van, or bus, are the proper child safety seats, booster seats, and seat belts used? Is there someone besides the driver supervising the children during transport?
- **Consistency.** Are the program's policies on meals, discipline, and issues such as toilet training the same as yours? How long have the staff worked at the center? How much experience do they have with children of your child's age?
- **Backup plans.** What happens if your child is sick or the child care program is closed?
- **Fees and services.** What is the cost? How are payments made? Are there other services available in addition to child care? Do these cost extra?
- **References.** Ask for references and contact information from parents who use the program, as well as at least 1 parent whose child was in the program during the past year.
- **Communication.** Can you talk with staff on a regular basis? If there was something sensitive you needed to bring up, would you feel comfortable talking to them?

Family child care

This type of care takes place in the caregiver's home. Many family child care providers have young children of their own. They may care for children who are the same age as their own children or for children of different ages.

Things to discuss

Before choosing family child care, talk with the provider about the following:

- **Others in the home.** Who lives in or visits the home (children, teens, and adults)? Are they family, what are their backgrounds, and how may they interact with your child?
- **Number of children.** What is the total number of children being cared for? The American Academy of Pediatrics (AAP) recommends that a family child care home should not have more than 6 children per adult caregiver, including the caregiver's own children. (Some states allow more children when at least 2 adults are available at all times in larger family child care homes.) The total number of children should be fewer when infants and toddlers are included. No caregiver who works alone should care for more than 2 children younger than 2 years.
- **Other caregivers.** Does the caregiver plan to leave the home during the day to run to the store or to drive children to school? If so, find out what the plan is for who will care for your child during this time.
- **Backup.** Because there usually is only 1 adult, backup care in an emergency situation must be nearby. In some areas, caregivers belong to a network of family child care providers who may provide training, shared toys, and backup help.
- **Qualifications.** Look for caregivers who are licensed or registered with the state. These caregivers will have unannounced visits by an inspector. Some family child care providers have earned accreditation as well.

In-home care

This is when the caregiver comes into or lives in your home. For many families, this is very convenient because caregivers often can arrange their schedules to match your needs. Because your child stays at home he does not have to adjust to a new setting. Your child may also be exposed to fewer illnesses because he will not be with groups of children. He may receive more individual attention, especially if the caregiver's main job is to care for your child. This type of caregiver is not monitored or supervised, and there is no formal licensure or regulation process.

Things to discuss

Before choosing in-home child care, talk with the provider about the following:

- **Your child's schedule.** Include such things as typical mealtimes, hand washing, toilet training, teeth brushing, and nap time.
- **Activities.** Discuss reading, playtime, and fun ways to be active inside and outside. Be sure to talk about what types of outings are acceptable for your child.
- **Discipline.** Let your caregiver know what types of discipline you approve of and what rules and limits you have set for your child.
- **Duties.** Write down and review what the caregiver will and will not do in your home. If your caregiver will also have housekeeping duties, stress that your child's needs must come first.
- **Safety.** Be sure your caregiver knows how to use the proper car safety seat, booster seat, or seat belt for your child. Also, talk about what you expect the caregiver to do in an emergency. Give your caregiver important phone numbers in case you cannot be reached.

> ### A checklist to help rate your choice
>
> "Is This the Right Place for My Child? 38 Research-Based Indicators of High-Quality Child Care" is a checklist put together by the National Association of Child Care Resource & Referral Agencies (NACCRRA) that you can use to evaluate child care programs. This checklist is on the NACCRRA Web site at www.naccrra.org/parent and available through a link from the AAP Web site www.healthychildcare.org. All of the questions are based on research about what is important to your child's health, safety, and development.

- **Limits.** Let your caregiver know how long your child is allowed to watch TV or videos or play computer games or other media. The AAP does not recommend TV for children younger than 2 years. For older children, the AAP recommends no more than 1 to 2 hours per day of educational, nonviolent programming.
- **Contact.** Be sure your caregiver knows how and when to contact you with questions or concerns.
- **Feedback.** The caregiver should give you a daily report of what occurred. Also, arrange for frequent, unannounced visits by a friend or family member who can observe how the caregiver interacts with your child.
- **Backup.** Be sure you have a backup plan for times when the caregiver is sick, needs time off, or goes on vacation. In some areas, child care resource and referral agencies or other community organizations can give you names of temporary in-home caregivers.

Different children, different care

Finding programs and caregivers to meet the needs of children with disabilities or other special needs can be challenging. Your child's doctor can help you and your child's caregiver plan for your child's special needs, development, activities, health, safety, and any problems that come up while you are using child care.

Planning for child care costs

Child care can be expensive, so families must budget ahead of time. While the cost may seem high, think about how little the caregiver is actually earning per hour for the responsibility of caring for your child. Be sure to budget for your backup care during those times when your child or caregiver is ill. You may qualify for state subsidies or assistance from your employer. Ask about

- Direct payment through cafeteria plans
- Dependent-care spending accounts (tax savings)
- Voucher programs
- Employer discounts

High-quality child care is a critical investment for your child. When care is consistent, developmentally sound, and emotionally supportive, there is a positive effect on the child and family. In some areas your local child care resource and referral agency can help you find licensed child care or apply for subsidies. For more information, visit www.naccrra.org or www.childcareaware.org.

Preparing your child

Most infants, up to 7 months of age, adjust well to good child care. Older infants may get upset when left with strangers. They will need extra time and your support to get to know the caregiver and to understand that you will pick them up at the end of the day. Starting new child care is often harder on the parents than it is on the child.

Being prepared makes any new experience easier. You can help your child adjust to a new child care arrangement. Try the following:

- Arrange a visit with in-home caregivers while you are at home or when you need child care for a short time.
- Visit the center or home with your child before beginning care. Show your child that you like and trust the caregiver.
- Check with the caregiver or center staff about the best time of the month or year for children to begin attending the program.
- Allow your child to carry a reminder of home to child care. A family photograph or small toy can be helpful.
- Talk with your child about child care and the caregiver.
- Read books about child care. (Check with your local library.)

Sudden changes in caregivers may be upsetting to a child. This can happen even if the new caregiver is kind and competent. You may want to arrange a meeting with the new caregiver or ask your child's doctor for advice. Parents need to help caregivers and the child deal with any changes in the child's routine at home or child care.

When your child gets sick

Children sometimes get sick or are injured while in child care. Talk with your child's caregiver in advance so that you both know what to expect and are prepared. Make sure that your caregiver can always reach you. Confirm a plan for emergency care in advance.

Many times, mildly ill children are allowed to stay with their caregiver as long as they can participate in most of the activities and don't require more care than their caregiver can provide. If the child needs extra rest, there must be a place for her to rest and still be observed.

Sometimes children need medicine while they are at child care. Every state and program will have different rules about what is allowed. Both prescription and over-the-counter medicines should be labeled with the child's name, dosage, and expiration date. The caregiver should have the parent's written permission to give the medicine, know how to give it safely, and properly record each dose. Depending on the regulations in your state, sometimes a doctor's note or instructions are required.

Resources

The following is a list of early education and child care resources. Check with your child's doctor or local child care resource and referral agency for resources in your community.

Web sites

AAP Early Education and Child Care Initiatives

This AAP site has a useful parent section and links to all the other Web sites listed here.
888/227-5409
www.healthychildcare.org

Child Care Aware (a program of NACCRRA)

800/424-2246
www.childcareaware.org

Healthy Kids, Healthy Care (provided by the National Resource Center for Health and Safety in Child Care and Early Education [NRC])

www.healthykids.us

National Association of Child Care Resource & Referral Agencies (NACCRRA)

703/341-4100
www.naccrra.org

National Association for the Education of Young Children

800/424-2460
www.naeyc.org

National Association for Family Child Care

800/359-3817
www.nafcc.org

National Resource Center for Health and Safety in Child Care and Early Education (NRC)

800/598-KIDS (800/598-5437)
http://nrckids.org

Books from the American Academy of Pediatrics

- *Caring for Our Children: National Health and Safety Performance Standards: Guidelines for Out-of-Home Child Care Programs, 2nd Edition*
- *Caring for Your Baby and Young Child: Birth to Age 5*
- *Caring for Your School-Age Child: Ages 5 to 12*
- *Managing Infectious Diseases in Child Care and Schools: A Quick Reference Guide*

Please note: Listing of resources does not imply an endorsement by the American Academy of Pediatrics (AAP). The AAP is not responsible for the content of the resources mentioned in this publication. Phone numbers and Web site addresses are as current as possible, but may change at any time.

The information contained in this publication should not be used as a substitute for the medical care and advice of your pediatrician. There may be variations in treatment that your pediatrician may recommend based on individual facts and circumstances.

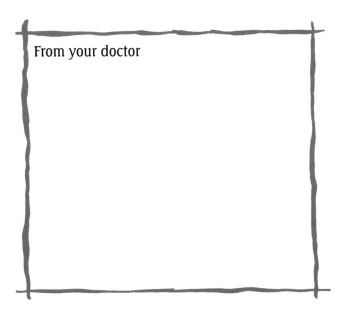

From your doctor

American Academy
of Pediatrics

DEDICATED TO THE HEALTH OF ALL CHILDREN™

The American Academy of Pediatrics is an organization of 60,000 primary care pediatricians, pediatric medical subspecialists, and pediatric surgical specialists dedicated to the health, safety, and well-being of infants, children, adolescents, and young adults.

American Academy of Pediatrics
Web site — www.aap.org

Copyright © 2007
American Academy of Pediatrics, Updated 11/07

Glossary

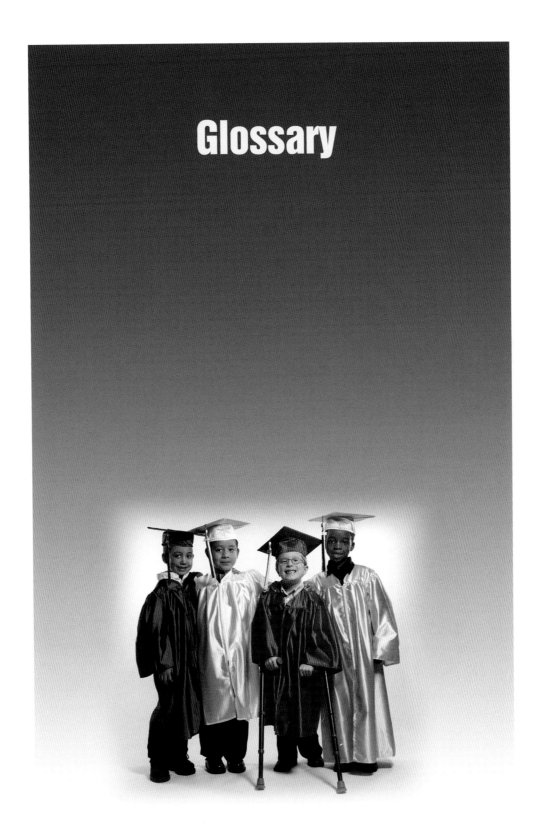

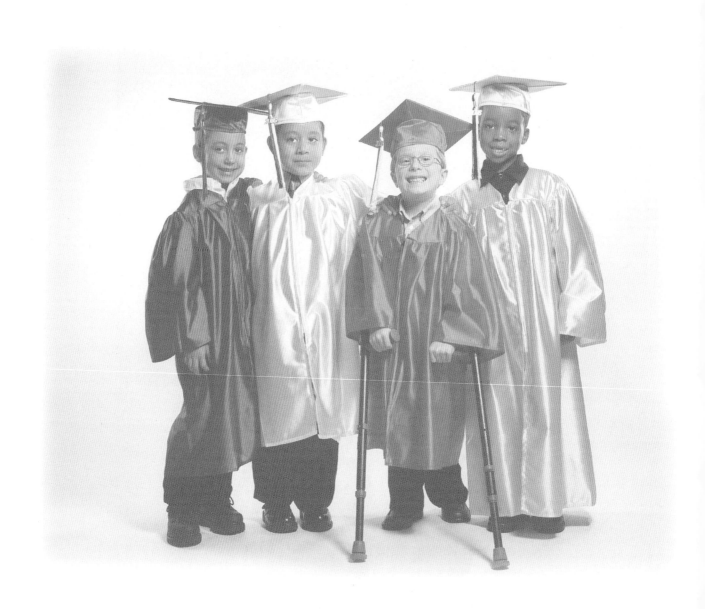

Glossary

These definitions are adapted from American Academy of Pediatrics, American Public Health Association, National Resource Center for Health and Safety in Child Care and Early Education. *Caring for Our Children: National Health and Safety Performance Standards: Guidelines for Out-of-Home Child Care Programs.* 2nd ed. Elk Grove Village, IL: American Academy of Pediatrics; 2002. Available at: http://nrckids.org/CFOC/index.html. Accessed September 17, 2010

AAP: Abbreviation for the American Academy of Pediatrics, a national organization of pediatricians founded in 1930 and dedicated to the improvement of child health and welfare.

Acute: Adjective describing an illness that has a sudden onset and is of short duration.

Allergen: A substance (eg, food, pollen, pets, mold, medication) that causes an allergic reaction.

Anaphylaxis: An allergic reaction to a specific allergen (eg, food, pollen, pets, mold, medication) that causes dangerous and potentially fatal complications, including swelling and closure of the airway that can lead to an inability to breathe.

Antibiotic prophylaxis: Antibiotics that are prescribed to *prevent* infections in infants and children in situations associated with an increased risk of serious infection with a specific disease. Usually prescribed in a low dose over a long period.

APHA: Abbreviation for the American Public Health Association, a national organization of health professionals that protects and promotes the health of the public through education, research, advocacy, and policy development.

Bleach solution: For sanitizing environmental surfaces—use a spray solution of a quarter (¼) cup of household liquid chlorine bleach (sodium hypochlorite) in 1 gallon of water, prepared fresh daily. Where blood contamination is likely, the concentration of bleach solution should be increased to 1 part bleach to 10 parts water because if hepatitis B virus is present in the blood, this higher concentration of bleach is required to kill it. See also *Disinfect.*

Body fluids: Urine, feces, saliva, blood, nasal discharge, eye discharge, and injury or tissue discharge.

Care Plan: A document that provides specific health care information, including any medications, procedures, precautions, or adaptations to diet or environment that may be needed to care for a child with chronic medical conditions or special health care needs. Care Plans also describe signs and symptoms of impending illness and outline the response needed to those signs and symptoms. A Care Plan is completed by a health care professional and should be updated on a regular basis.

Caregiver: Used in this book to indicate the primary staff who work directly with children in child care centers, small or large family child care homes, or schools (ie, director, teacher, aide, child care provider, or those with other titles or child contact roles).

Catheterization: The process of inserting a hollow tube into an organ of the body, for an investigative purpose or to give some form of treatment (eg, remove urine from the bladder of a child with neurologic disease).

CDC: Abbreviation for the Centers for Disease Control and Prevention, which is responsible for monitoring communicable diseases, immunization status, injuries, and congenital malformations, and performing other disease and injury surveillance activities in the United States.

Center: A facility that provides care and education for any number of children in a nonresidential setting and is open on a regular basis (it is not a drop-in facility).

Children with special health care needs: Children who have or are at increased risk for a chronic physical, developmental, behavioral, or emotional condition and who also require health and related services of a type or amount beyond that required by children generally.

Chronic: Adjective describing an infection or illness that lasts a long time (months or years).

Clean: To remove dirt and debris (eg, blood, urine, feces) by scrubbing and washing with a detergent solution and rinsing with water.

CPR: Abbreviation for cardiopulmonary resuscitation, emergency measures performed by a person on another person whose breathing or heart activity has stopped. Measures include closed-chest cardiac compressions and mouth-to-mouth ventilation in a regular sequence.

Disinfect: To eliminate virtually all germs from inanimate surfaces by using chemicals (eg, products registered with the US Environmental Protection Agency as "disinfectants") or physical agents (eg, heat).

Educator: A teacher or caregiver who is professionally responsible for the education of the children who are placed in his or her care.

Emergency response practices: Procedures used to call for emergency medical assistance, reach parents or emergency contacts, arrange for transfer to medical assistance, and render first aid to the injured person.

Exclusion: Denying admission of an ill child or staff member to a facility or asking the child or staff member to leave if present.

Facility: A legal definition of the buildings, grounds, equipment, and people involved in providing child care or education of any type.

Febrile: The condition of having an abnormally high body temperature (fever), often as a response to infection.

Fever: An elevation of body temperature. Body temperature can be elevated by overheating caused by overdressing or a hot environment, reactions to medications, inflammatory conditions (eg, arthritis, lupus), cancers, and response to infection. For this purpose, fever is defined as temperature above 101°F (38.3°C) orally, above 102°F (38.9°C) rectally, or of 100°F (37.8°C) or higher taken axillary (armpit) or measured by any equivalent method. Fever is an indication of the body's response to something, but is neither a disease nor a serious problem by itself.

Gastric tube feeding: The administration of nourishment through a tube that has been surgically inserted directly into the stomach.

Gestational: Occurring during or related to pregnancy.

Gross-motor skills: Large movements involving the arms, legs, feet, or entire body (eg, crawling, running, jumping).

Group care setting: A facility where children from more than one family receive care together.

Health care professional: Someone who practices medicine with or without supervision, and who is licensed by an established body. The most common types of health care professionals include physicians, nurse practitioners, nurses, and physician assistants.

Health consultant: A physician, a certified pediatric or family nurse practitioner, a registered nurse, or an environmental, an oral, a mental health, a nutrition, or another health professional who has pediatric and child care experience and is knowledgeable in pediatric health practice, child care, licensing, and community resources. The health consultant provides guidance and assistance to child care staff on health aspects of the facility.

HIV: Abbreviation for human immunodeficiency virus.

Immunity: The body's ability to fight a particular infection. Immunity can come from antibodies (immune globulin), cells, or other factors.

Immunizations: Vaccines that are given to children and adults to help them develop protection (antibodies) against specific infections. Vaccines may contain an inactivated or a killed agent, part of the agent, an inactivated toxin made by an agent (toxoid), or a weakened live organism.

Individualized Education Program (IEP): A written document, derived from Part B of the Individuals With Disabilities Education Act, that is designed to meet a child's individual educational program needs. The main purposes of an IEP are to set reasonable learning goals and state the services that the school district will provide for a child with special educational needs. Every child who is qualified for special educational services provided by the school is required to have an IEP.

Individualized Family Service Plan (IFSP): A written document, derived from Part C of the Individuals With Disabilities Education Act, that is formulated in collaboration with the family to meet the needs of a child with a developmental disability or delay; assist the family in its care for a child's educational, therapeutic, and health needs; and deal with the family's needs to the extent to which the family wishes assistance.

Infant: A child between the time of birth and 12 months of age.

Infection: A condition caused by the multiplication of an infectious agent in the body.

Lead agency: Refers to an individual state choice for the agency that will receive and allocate federal and state funding for children with special educational needs. Federal funding is allocated to individual states in accordance with the Individuals With Disabilities Education Act.

Lethargy: Unusual sleepiness or low activity level.

Mainstreaming: A widely used term that describes the philosophy and activities associated with providing services to persons with disabilities in community settings, especially in school programs, where such children or other persons are integrated with persons without disabilities and are entitled to attend programs and have access to all services available in the community.

Medications: Any substances that are intended to diagnose, cure, treat, or prevent disease, or affect the structure or function of the body of humans or other animals.

Nasogastric tube feeding: The administration of nourishment using a plastic tube that stretches from the nose to the stomach.

Nonprescription medications: Drugs that are generally regarded as safe for use if the label directions and warnings are followed. Nonprescription medications are also called over-the-counter drugs because they can be purchased without a prescription from a health care professional. Foods or cosmetics that are intended to treat or prevent disease or affect the functions of the human body (eg, suntan lotion, fluoride toothpaste, antiperspirant deodorants, anti-dandruff shampoo) are also considered to be nonprescription medications.

Occupational therapy: Treatment based on the use of occupational activities of a typical child (eg, play, feeding, toileting, dressing). Child-specific exercises are developed to encourage a child with mental or physical disabilities to contribute to his or her own recovery and development.

OSHA: Abbreviation for the Occupational Safety and Health Administration of the US Department of Labor, which regulates health and safety in the workplace.

Parent: The child's natural or adoptive mother or father, guardian, or other legally responsible person.

Pediatric first aid: Emergency care and treatment of an injured child before definite medical and surgical management can be secured. Pediatric first aid includes rescue breathing and addressing choking.

Physical therapy: The use of physical agents and methods (eg, massage, therapeutic exercises, hydrotherapy, electrotherapy) to assist a child with physical or mental disabilities to optimize his or her individual physical development or restore his or her normal body function after illness or injury.

Prenatal: Existing or occurring before birth (as in prenatal medical care).

Primary care provider (PCP): The physician in the child's medical home who supervises the team that provides preventive care, routine illness care, and care coordination with the child's specialists and therapists.

Reflux: An abnormal backward flow of liquids. The term is commonly used to describe gastroesophageal reflux of stomach contents into the esophagus, or urinary reflux of urine from the bladder up toward the kidneys.

Rescue breathing: The process of breathing air into the lungs of a person who has stopped breathing. This process is also called artificial respiration.

Sanitize: To remove filth or soil and small amounts of certain bacteria. For an inanimate surface to be considered sanitary, the surface must be clean (see *Clean*) and the number of germs must be reduced to such a level that disease transmission by that surface is unlikely. This procedure is less rigorous than disinfection (see *Disinfect*) and is applicable to a wide variety of routine housekeeping procedures involving, for example, bedding, bathrooms, kitchen countertops, floors, and walls.

Seizure: A sudden attack or convulsion caused by involuntary, uncontrolled bursts of electrical activity in the brain that can result in a wide variety of clinical manifestations, including muscle twitches, staring, tongue biting, loss of consciousness, and total body shaking.

Staff: Used here to indicate all personnel employed at the child care facility or school, including caregivers, teachers, and personnel who do not provide direct care to children (eg, cooks, drivers, housekeeping personnel).

Standard precautions: Techniques used to protect a person when there is contact with non-intact skin, mucous membranes, blood, all body fluids, and excretions except sweat. The general methods of infection prevention are indicated for all people in the group care setting and are designed to reduce the risk of transmission of microorganisms from recognized and unrecognized sources of infection. Although standard precautions were designed to apply to hospital settings, except for the use of masks and gowns, they also apply in group care settings. Standard precautions involve use of barriers (eg, gloves) as well as hand washing, and cleaning and sanitizing surfaces. Group care adaptation of standard precautions (exceptions from the use in hospital settings) are as follows:
- Use of nonporous gloves is optional except when blood or blood-containing body fluids may be involved.
- Gowns and masks are not required.
- Appropriate barriers include materials, such as disposable diaper table paper and disposable towels and surfaces, that can be sanitized in group care settings.

Substitute staff: Caregivers/teachers who are hired for one day or an extended period but are not considered permanent workers in their assigned positions.

Toddler: A child between the age of ambulation and toilet learning and training (usually between 13 and 35 months).

Universal precautions: A term used by OSHA that applies to protection against blood and other body fluids that contain blood, semen, and vaginal secretions, but not to feces, nasal secretions, sputum, sweat, tears, urine, saliva, and vomitus, unless they contain visible blood or are likely to contain blood. Universal precautions include avoiding injuries that are caused by sharp instruments or devices and the use of protective barriers, such as gloves, gowns, aprons, masks, or protective eyewear, that can reduce the risk of exposure of the worker's skin or mucous membranes that could come in contact with materials that may contain blood-borne pathogens while the worker is providing first aid or care.

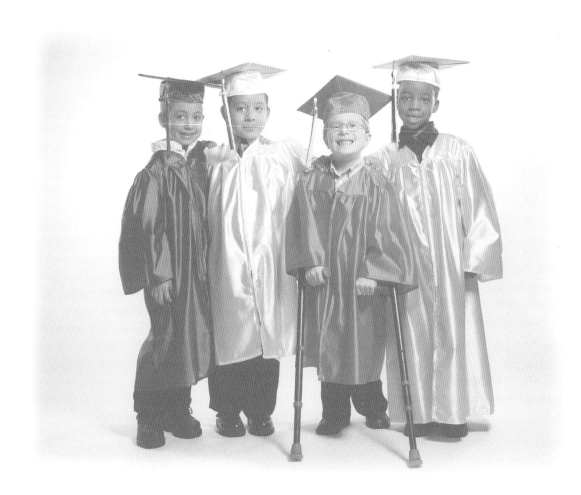

Additional Resources

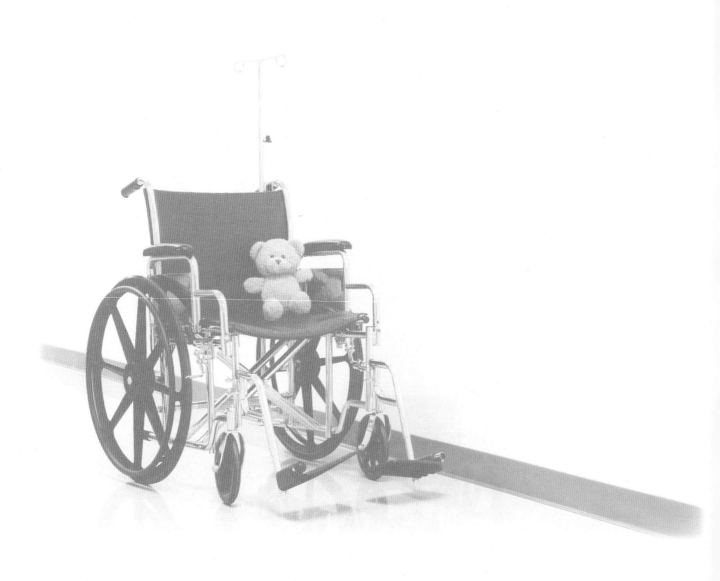

Additional Resources

General Resources

This is a guide to key resources that supplement the content of this book.

Books

- American Academy of Pediatrics. *Managing Infectious Diseases in Child Care and Schools: A Quick Reference Guide.* Aronson SS, Shope TR, eds. 2nd ed. Elk Grove Village, IL: American Academy of Pediatrics; 2009
- American Academy of Pediatrics. *Pediatric First Aid for Caregivers and Teachers.* Rev ed. Sudbury, MA: Jones and Bartlett Publishers; 2007
- American Academy of Pediatrics. *School Health: Policy & Practice.* 6th ed. Elk Grove Village, IL: American Academy of Pediatrics; 2004
- American Academy of Pediatrics, American Public Health Association, National Resource Center for Health and Safety in Child Care and Early Education. *Caring for Our Children: National Health and Safety Performance Standards: Guidelines for Out-of-Home Child Care Programs.* 2nd ed. Elk Grove Village, IL: American Academy of Pediatrics; 2002. Available at: http://nrckids.org/CFOC/index.html. Accessed September 17, 2010
- Taras H, Duncan P, Luckenbill D, Robinson J, Wheeler L, Wooley S, eds. *Health, Mental Health, and Safety Guidelines for Schools.* Elk Grove Village, IL: American Academy of Pediatrics; 2004

American Academy of Pediatrics Policy Statements

These and other pertinent American Academy of Pediatrics policy statements can be accessed at www.aappolicy.org.

- American Academy of Pediatrics, Committee on School Health. Guidelines for the administration of medication in school. *Pediatrics.* 2003;112:697–699
- American Academy of Pediatrics, Council on School Health. Medical emergencies occurring at school. *Pediatrics.* 2008;122:887–894
- American Academy of Pediatrics, Council on School Health. Role of the school nurse in providing school health services. *Pediatrics.* 2008;121:1052–1056

Topical Resources

Selected resources and references that apply specifically to chapters within this publication are as follows:

Chapter 2: Background

References

- Sokal-Gutierrez K. *Child Care and Children with Special Needs: A Training Manual for Early Childhood Professionals.* Newark, DE: Video Active Productions; 2001
- Szabo JL. Maddie's story: inclusion through physical and occupational therapy. *Teach Except Child.* 2000;33:12–18
- US Department of Education. Assistance to states for the education of children with disabilities and the early intervention program for infants and toddlers with disabilities; final regulations. *Fed Regist.* 1999;64:12406–12672
- US Department of Education. *To Assure the Free Appropriate Public Education of All Children With Disabilities (Individuals With Disabilities Education Act, Section 618): Twenty-first Annual Report to Congress on the Implementation of the Individuals With Disabilities Education Act.* Washington, DC: Department of Education; 1999
- Wright PWD, Wright PD. *Wrightslaw: From Emotions to Advocacy: The Special Education Survival Guide.* 2nd ed. Hartfield, VA: Harbor House Law Press; 2006

Resources

National Dissemination Center for Children with Disabilities, 800/695-0285 (voice/TTY), www.nichcy.org, has several publications that discuss special education services and what is involved when a child is evaluated.

- *Questions and Answers about IDEA: Purposes and Key Definitions* (www.nichcy.org/InformationResources/Documents/NICHCY%20PUBS/QA1.pdf)
- *Questions and Answers about IDEA: Parent Participation* (www.nichcy.org/InformationResources/Documents/NICHCY%20PUBS/QA2.pdf)
- *Questions Often Asked by Parents About Special Education Services* (www.nichcy.org/InformationResources/Documents/NICHCY%20PUBS/lg1.pdf)
- *Your Child's Evaluation,* 2nd Edition (www.nichcy.org/InformationResources/Documents/NICHCY%20PUBS/bp1.pdf)

Chapter 5: Special Care Plan Implementation Strategies for Caregivers/Teachers

Resources

- Child Care Aware, www.childcareaware.org
- Child Care Law Center, www.childcarelaw.org
- Healthy Child Care Consultant Network Support Center, http://hcccnsc.edc.org
- National Association of Child Care Resource & Referral Agencies, www.naccrra.org
- Technical Assistance Alliance for Parent Centers, www.taalliance.org

Training Resources

- American Academy of Pediatrics, www.aap.org
- California Childcare Health Program, www.ucsfchildcarehealth.org
- Healthy Child Care America, www.healthychildcare.org
- Healthy Child Care Pennsylvania, www.ecels-healthychildcarepa.org
- Healthy Kids, Healthy Care, www.healthykids.us
- National Association for the Education of Young Children, www.naeyc.org
- National Resource Center for Health and Safety in Child Care and Early Education, http://nrckids.org
- National Training Institute for Child Care Health Consultants, http://nti.unc.edu

Chapter 6: Medication Administration Issues

References

- American Academy of Pediatrics. *School Health: Policy & Practice.* 6th ed. Elk Grove Village, IL: American Academy of Pediatrics; 2004
- American Academy of Pediatrics, American Public Health Association, National Resource Center for Health and Safety in Child Care and Early Education. *Medication Administration. Applicable Standards from: Caring for Our Children: National Health and Safety Performance Standards: Guidelines for Out-of-Home Child Care Programs.* 2nd ed. Elk Grove Village, IL: American Academy of Pediatrics; 2003. Available at: http://nrckids.org/SPINOFF/MED/Medication.pdf. Accessed June 24, 2009
- American Academy of Pediatrics, Committee on School Health. Guidelines for the administration of medication in school. *Pediatrics.* 2003;112:697–699

- Association for Children of New Jersey. *Ensuring Safe Medication Administration to Children in New Jersey's Child Care Programs.* May 2006. Available at: http://www.acnj.org/admin.asp?uri=2081&action=15&di=820&ext=pdf&view=yes. Accessed June 24, 2009
- Catenzaro SA. *Issues and Barriers to Medication Administration in Child Care Centers* [master's thesis]. New Haven, CT: Yale University School of Nursing, New Haven; 2001
- Connecticut Nurses' Association, Healthy Child Care Connecticut. *Medication Administration Training Program.* Meriden, CT: Connecticut Nurses' Association; 2005
- Heschel RT, Crowley AA, Cohen SS. State policies regarding nursing delegation and medication administration in child care settings: a case study. *Policy Polit Nurs Pract.* 2005;6:86–98
- National Association for Regulatory Administration, National Child Care Information and Technical Assistance Center. *The 2005 Child Care Licensing Study: Final Report.* Available at: http://nara.affiniscape.com/associations/4734/files/2005%20Licensing%20Study%20Final%20Report_Web.pdf. Accessed June 24, 2009
- National Association of School Nurses. *Medication Administration in the School Setting.* Scarborough, ME: National Association of School Nurses; 2003

Resources

- American Academy of Pediatrics, www.aap.org
- American Nurses Association, www.nursingworld.org
- Connecticut Department of Public Health, Child Day Care Licensing Program, http://www.ct.gov/dph/cwp/view.asp?a=3141&Q=387158
- Connecticut Nurses' Association, Medication Administration Training Program, http://www.ctnurses.org/displaycommon.cfm?an=1&subarticlenbr=43
- Head Start Program Performance Standards, http://eclkc.ohs.acf.hhs.gov/hslc/Program%20Design%20and%20Management/Head%20Start%20Requirements/Head%20Start%20Requirements
- Healthy Child Care America, www.healthychildcare.org
- Healthy Child Care Ohio, www.coadinc.org/Main.php?page=programs-ece-health-safety
- Healthy Child Care Pennsylvania, www.ecels-healthychildcarepa.org

- Medication Administration in Child Care, Specialized Trainings and the Quality Point for the Revised Rated License, www.childcarehealthtraining.org/epr/PDF/Quality_Point_Clarification.pdf
- National Association for the Education of Young Children, Early Childhood Program Standards, www.naeyc.org
- National Association of Pediatric Nurse Practitioners, www.napnap.org
- National Resource Center for Health and Safety in Child Care and Early Education, http://nrckids.org
- National Training Institute for Child Care Health Consultants, http://nti.unc.edu
- New York State Office of Children & Family Services, www.ocfs.state.ny.us/main
- Qualistar Early Learning, Medication Administration Training, www.qualistar.org/professionals/mat.php
- Virginia Department of Social Services, Medication Administration Training, https://www.dss.virginia.gov/family/cc_providertrain/mat/index.cgi

Chapter 8: Planning for Emergencies

Resources

- American Academy of Pediatrics Children & Disasters, www.aap.org/disasters
- American Academy of Pediatrics policy statements
  - ~ American Academy of Pediatrics, Committee on Pediatric Emergency Medicine, Committee on Medical Liability, Task Force on Terrorism. The pediatrician and disaster preparedness. *Pediatrics.* 2006;117:560–565
  - ~ American Academy of Pediatrics, Committee on Pediatric Emergency Medicine. Preparation for emergencies in the offices of pediatricians and pediatric primary care providers. *Pediatrics.* 2007;120:200–212
  - ~ American Academy of Pediatrics, Council on School Health. Medical emergencies occurring at school. *Pediatrics.* 2008;122:887–894
  - ~ American Academy of Pediatrics, Council on School Health. Disaster planning for schools. *Pediatrics.* 2008;122:895–901
- Pediatric First Aid for Caregivers and Teachers Online, http://pedfactsonline.com

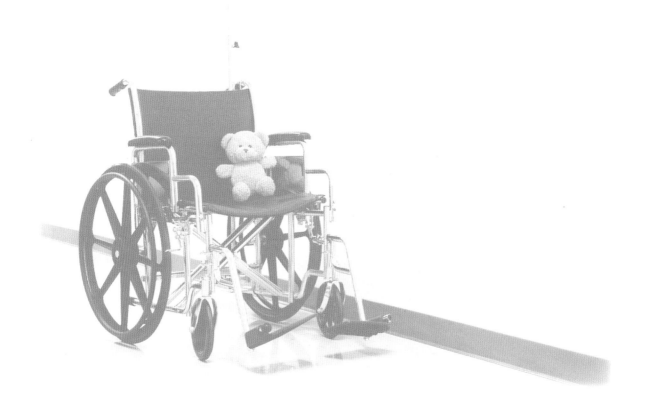

Index

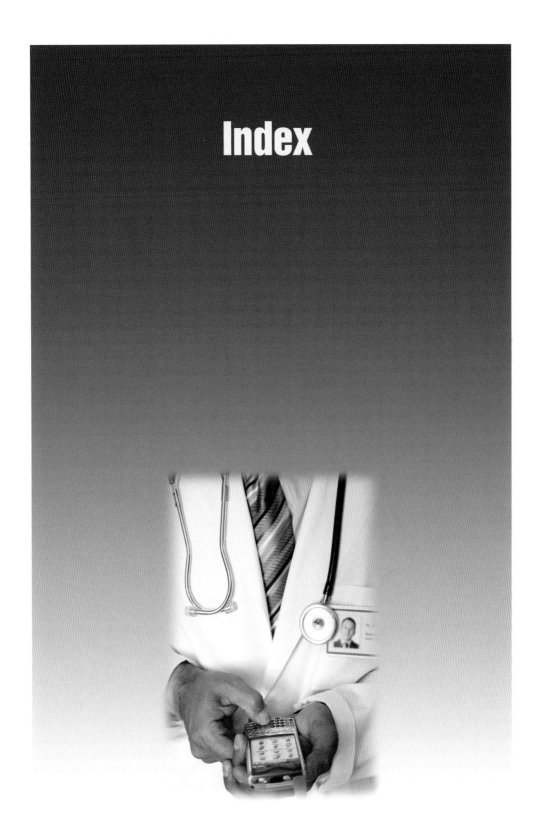

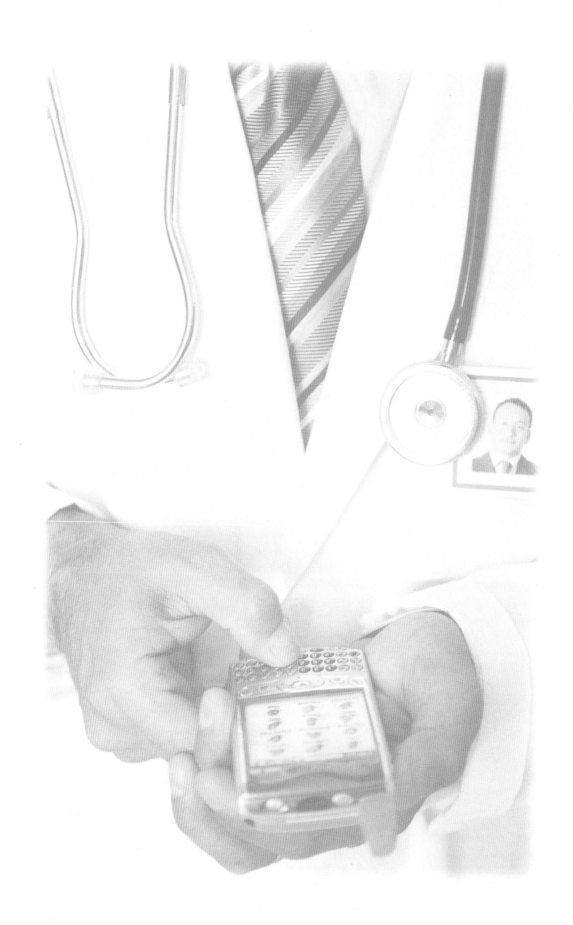

Index

A

Functional heart conditions, 99
Furosemide (Lasix), 106

G

Galactosemia, 129
Gastroenterologists, 17
Gastroesophageal reflux disease (GERD), 91–92
  apnea and, 119
  characteristics of children with, 91
  defined, 91
  dietary considerations for, 91
  as emergency, 91
  medications for, 91
  physical environment for, 91
  resources on, 92
  statistics on, 91
  training or policies for, 92
Gastrointestinal system in premature newborns, 120
Gastrostomy tubes, 93–94
  defined, 93
  dietary considerations for, 94
  elements of Care Plan for, 93–94
  as emergency, 94
  physical environment for, 94
  resources on, 94
  statistics on, 93
  training or policies for, 94
  treatment team for, 93
Generalized seizures, 125
Geneticists, 17
Glomerulonephritis. *See* Nephritis (glomerulonephritis)
Glucagon, 87
Gluten, 77
Gluten-free diet, 77
  resources on, 78
Gluten Intolerance Group of North America, 78
Gluten-sensitive enteropathy. *See* Celiac disease (gluten-sensitive enteropathy)
Grand mal seizures, 125

H

Haberman Feeder, 82
Hands & Voices, 97
Head Start Performance Standards, 33
Health care professionals
  as member of core team, 15
  responsibilities for Care Plan, 22
Health consultants
  ongoing support by, 36
  role of, 16
Health Insurance Portability and Accountability Act (HIPAA), 23, 30
  consent form to obtain privacy-protected information for physician or primary health care provider, 157
Hearing in premature newborns, 120
Hearing loss, 95–97
  for babies with cleft lip and cleft palate, 81
  Care Plan for, 96
  characteristics of children, 95–96
  defined, 95

elements of Care Plan for, 96
  medications for, 96
  physical environment for, 96
  resources on, 97
  statistics on, 95
  training or policies for, 97
  treatment team for, 96
  types of, 95
Heart conditions, 99–103
  arrhythmia as, 102
  cardiomyopathy as, 103
  characteristics of children with functional, 101
  defined, 99
  hypertension as, 103
  Kawasaki disease as, 101–102
Heart defects, structural, 105–106
Heart failure, 99
Heart murmur, 99
Heart palpitations, 102
Hematologists, 17, 73
Hemophilia, 73
Hepatitis, 107–108
  characteristics of children with, 107
  defined, 107
  dietary considerations for, 107–108
  as emergency, 108
  medications for, 107
  physical environment for, 108
  resources on, 108
  statistics on, 107
  training or policies for, 108
  treatment team for, 107
Hepatitis A, 107
Hepatitis B, 73, 107
Hepatitis C, 73, 107
High blood pressure. *See* Hypertension (high blood pressure)
High blood sugar, 87
Hives (urticaria), 53, 54
Homocystinuria, 129
Human Growth Foundation, 52
Human immunodeficiency virus (HIV), 73, 109–110
  characteristics of children with, 109
  defined, 109
  as emergency, 110
  medications for, 109
  physical environment for, 109–110
  resources on, 110
  statistics on, 109
  training or policies for, 110
  treatment team for, 109
Hydrocephalus or shunts, 111–112, 131
  characteristics of children with, 111
  defined, 111
  as emergency, 111–112
  physical environment for, 111
  resources on, 112
  training or policies for, 112
  treatment team for, 111
Hydronephrosis, 116

N

O